Ethical Dilemmas
and Nursing Practice

third edition

Ethical Dilemmas and Nursing Practice

third edition

Anne J. Davis, RN, PhD, FAAN
Professor
School of Nursing
University of California
San Francisco, California

Mila A. Aroskar, RN, EdD, FAAN
Associate Professor
School of Public Health
University of Minnesota
Minneapolis, Minnesota

APPLETON & LANGE
Norwalk, Connecticut/San Mateo, California

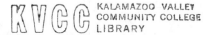

0-8385-2275-0

Copyright © 1991 by Appleton & Lange
A Publishing Division of Prentice Hall

Copyright © 1983, 1978 by Appleton-Century-Crofts

91 92 93 94 95 / 10 9 8 7 6 5 4 3 2 1

Prentice Hall International (UK) Limited, *London*
Prentice Hall of Australia Pty. Limited, *Sydney*
Prentice Hall Canada Inc., *Toronto*
Prentice Hall Hispanoamericana, S.A., *Mexico*
Prentice Hall of India Private Limited, *New Delhi*
Prentice Hall of Japan, Inc., *Tokyo*
Simon & Schuster Asia Pte. Ltd., *Singapore*
Editora Prentice Hall do Brasil, Ltda., *Rio de Janeiro*
Prentice Hall, *Englewood Cliffs, New Jersey*

Library of Congress Cataloging-in-Publication Data

Davis, Anne, J., 1931–
    Ethical dilemmas and nursing practice / Anne J. Davis, Mila A. Aroskar. — 3rd ed.
        p. cm.
    Includes bibliographical references.
    Includes index.
    ISBN 0-8385-2275-0
    1. Nursing ethics.   2. Medical ethics.   I. Aroskar, Mila A.
II. Title.
    [DNLM: 1. Ethics, Nursing.   WY 85 C261e]
RT85.D33   1991
174'.2—dc20
DNLM/DLC   90-14517
for Library of Congress   CIP

Acquisitions Editor: Marion Kalstein-Welch
Production Editor: James J. Gormley
Designer: Janice Barsevich

PRINTED IN THE UNITED STATES OF AMERICA

Contributors

Marsha Fowler, RN, PhD
Professor
School of Nursing
Graduate School of Theology
Azusa Pacific University
Azusa, California

Sara Fry, RN, PhD, FAAN
Associate Professor
School of Nursing
University of Maryland
Baltimore, Maryland

Contents

Preface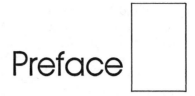

We wrote the first edition of this book in 1978 while we were Kennedy postdoctoral fellows at Harvard University. Since that first edition, a number of important developments have occurred. Ethics has become more central in teaching nursing students and in clinical nursing practice. Nonetheless, there is still room for improvement. Certainly more nursing ethics books are available, which makes the selection of materials more diverse and much richer. More research focused on nursing's ethical issues has been conducted.

In addition to these developments, ethical issues in health care have received more attention in the mass media. At times this attention has come from reports or legal decisions, as in the case of abortion and the right-to-die question. Clinical settings, with new acute care technology or long-term care issues, influenced by the increase in the elderly population and cost containment efforts, constitute a major arena for ethical dilemmas.

Since the first edition, the AIDS epidemic has raised crucial ethical questions, some of which society and health professionals continue to debate. Populations such as the homeless and others without health care insurance reinforce the ethical issues in health policies that stem from a declining system in crisis, and hold up to all of us fundamental questions about our shared humanity and the common good.

On the international scene, some areas of the world have experienced fundamental changes that have the potential to create a brighter future. Other areas have experienced economic and social tragedy. All of these events and changes have an impact on people's health and the health care system. Embedded in change of all types, we find questions of values, rights, and obligations. Concepts of individual rights and the common good present themselves for examination, debate, and solution. Within this international ferment, activities in nursing-ethics have continued to increase.

We have been most pleased with the response to this book. It is this response that has led us to prepare the third edition. We want to thank all those who assisted with this edition. Two colleagues, Marsha Fowler and Sara Fry, assisted us by updating two chapters. Vee Sutherland, who did a library search, was an answer to a prayer. Paul Blanchard and Hanna Regev typed the manuscript. The people at Appleton & Lange kept us on our toes in the editing process. To all of these colleagues, we acknowledge our thanks. We continue to appreciate the importance of ethical dilemmas confronting nurses and applaud the courage that nurses have demonstrated. This third edition is dedicated to them.

Anne J. Davis, RN, PhD, FAAN
Mila A. Aroskar, RN, EdD, FAAN

CHAPTER 1

Health Care Ethics and Ethical Dilemmas

ETHICS

Traditionally, philosophy, as a body of knowledge, has asked and attempted to answer in a formal and disciplined manner the great questions of life that any of us might raise with ourselves in our more reflective moments. The branch of philosophy called *ethics*, also referred to as moral philosophy, deals with important questions of human conduct that have great relevance to us as individuals and as health professionals. Ethics, as a body of knowledge, has evolved in the Western philosophical tradition since the Golden Age of Greece and deals with the concept of morality and with moral problems and judgments. Metaethics delineates the extent to which moral judgments are reasonable or otherwise justifiable, whereas normative ethics raises the question of what is right or what ought to be done in a situation that calls for a moral decision. It examines individual rights and obligations as well as the common good. Descriptive ethics focuses on what people actually do in given situations. Normative ethics and descriptive ethics are the frameworks for this book. While an ethic of virtue, which addresses the question of what sort of person should I be, is of utmost importance, it is not the focus here. Rather, the question of what ought I do in a given situation of ethical conflict provides the direction. What one does in action cannot always or easily be separated from the sort of person one is. Our purpose, however, is to focus on ethical reasoning and what a moral agent should take into account in that reasoning. In examining this book, the reader would do well to remember that Dante in his Divine Comedy maintained that the hottest places in hell are reserved for those who maintain their neutrality in times of great moral crises.

The word *ethics*, derived from the Greek term *ethos*, originally meant customs, habitual usages, conduct, and character, and the word *morals*, derived from the Latin *mores*, means customs or habit. Today, in the widest sense, these two words refer to conduct, character, and motives involved in moral acts and include the notion of approval or disapproval of a given conduct, character, or motive that we describe by such words as good, desirable, right, and worthy, or conversely by such words as bad, undesirable, wrong, evil, and unworthy. Often when we speak of the ethics or morals of an individual or group, we refer to a set of rules or body of principles. Each society, religion, and professional group has its principles or standards of conduct, and as persons concerned with being reasonable in our conduct, we rely on these standards for guidance. Not to seek guidance from such principles or rules would mean that most likely we would engage in unpredictable behavior and therefore would be considered unreliable, so that others could not count on us in daily social interaction.

In discussions on this topic, the word *ethics* often becomes synonymous with *morality*. Morality has been defined as a social enterprise and not just an invention or discovery of the individual for his own guidance. This social nature of morality is not limited to its being a system governing the relations of one person to others or one's code of action with respect to others. Obviously, morality is social in this sense, but also, and importantly, morality is social in its origins, sanctions, and functions, since we are born into a society that has developed and continues to maintain mores, laws, and ethical codes.[1] As a social system of regulations, morality shares some similarities with both the law and social convention or etiquette. Convention, as we usually define it, has to do with considerations of taste, appearance, and convenience, and does not deal with matters of crucial social importance. Convention and morality share similarities in that neither is created or changed by a deliberate judicial, legislative, or executive act; therefore physical force or the threat of it does not serve as a sanction. Verbal signs of approval or disapproval, praise or blame, become social sanctions in these instances. In its focus on crucial matters of social importance, such as individual and group rights and obligations, morality shares similarities with the law.[2]

Although a standard of conduct serves to guide our individual and societal morality, we can still face ethical dilemmas. Nurses confront many ethical dilemmas in their practice. Such dilemmas include whether to care for a so-called noncompliant patient,[3] decisions to discontinue intensive therapy,[4] keeping confidences,[5] patient advocacy,[6] refusing to care for a patient with acquired immunodeficiency syndrome (AIDS).[7] We may be ethical to the extent that our behavior elicits approval and respect from others; however, we still confront moral perplexity and moral doubt. For example, in a situation in which our ethical code guides us to tell the truth, we decide to withhold truthful information because we believe such knowledge will cause psychological harm to the individual hearing it. Such a situation confronts health professionals, particularly in caring for the terminally ill patient. This example shows that in honoring one moral principle we can violate another: If we tell the truth we may risk doing harm to the hearer. On the other hand, if we do not tell the truth, we violate the individual's right to knowledge that affects his self-determination. As one ethicist has said, the degree of confidence a community can have in its health professionals remains one critical consideration in the issue of truth telling, or veracity, in the health sciences.[8] Although a set of rules is vital to human conduct, it cannot be wholly depended upon for guidance, since it can never be complete enough to anticipate all possible occasions involving moral decisions. To be useful at all, moral principles must be general in nature, but this generality also inescapably makes their utility limited.

Socrates, the patron saint of moral philosophy, in the Crito dialogue argued that we must let reason determine our ethical decisions rather than emotion.[9] To accomplish this we must have factual information about the situation and keep our minds clear as we deliberate the issue. We need to be aware of our values and how they influence our definition of an ethical situation. In addition, values held in common by all nurses must be taken into account.[10] It is not enough to appeal to what people generally think, since they may be wrong, but we must, by informed reasoning, find an answer that we regard as correct. And importantly, according to Socrates, we ought never to do what is morally wrong. The proposal of what we should do in a situation must be viewed as to its rightness or wrongness as concluded after informed reasoning and not as to what will happen to us as a consequence, or what others will think of us, or how we feel about the situation. In his arguments, Socrates appealed to a general moral rule or principle that, after reflection, he accepted as valid and applicable to particular situations. But in addition, Socrates, aware of the fact that sometimes two or more moral rules apply to the same case but do not lead to the same conclusion, resolved this conflict by determining which rules take precedence over others. Here he went beyond simply appealing to rules, since they conflict with one another, and established what he called basic rules and derivative rules, which rest on the more basic ones. A reasoning process that establishes basic ethical rules leads to the inevitable question of how ethical principles and judgments are to be justified. A full-fledged discussion develops in moral philosophy when we pass beyond the stage in which we are directed only by traditional rules of conduct, which have limited application to complex ethical situations, and move to a stage where we think critically about an ethical dilemma in ways that allow us to use traditional rules as general principles coupled with ethical reasoning going beyond these traditional rules.

As has been indicated, not all ethical dilemmas can be resolved by an appeal to our common moral rules, and this fact lies at the center of moral philosophy as a field of inquiry. Let it be stressed, however, that the traditional interest in ethics as a subject matter must not be confused with the practical interest of moral beings. To avoid the mistake of supposing that a knowledge of moral theory is sufficient for the improvement of our moral practice, we must realize that the theoretical interest is concerned with knowing and the practical interest with doing.[11] A moralist engages in reflection and discussion about what is morally right or wrong, good or evil. A moral philosopher thinks and writes about the ways in which moral terms like *right* or *good* are used by moralists when they deliver their moral judgments.[12] If our object is to discover unambiguous answers to ethical dilemmas quickly and effortlessly, most likely we will be bewildered by the complexity of these dilemmas. Furthermore, we will most surely experience disappointment if we expect instant truth, for one does not mine ethical dilemmas as easily as one mines for diamonds, but a concern for ethical principles may prove to be the more valuable of the two endeavors.

HEALTH CARE ETHICS

Building on accumulated knowledge, especially from the seventeenth through the nineteenth centuries, advances in medical science and technology have progressed triumphantly during the twentieth century. In the wake of this progress, two sets of major problems related to optimal health care have arisen. The first set of problems concerns the adequate distribution and availability of health care and the second set concerns the danger of becoming so infatuated with the technological dimensions of health care that we cease to question their limitations. Specifically, we can unintentionally lose sight of the axiomatic foundation of health care, which is that human beings cannot be understood in mechanistic terms only. To do so, though, shows a limited view, a view that could violate that very foundation.

The health sciences make many demands upon the abilities, special training and character of their practitioners. One of the most basic of these demands requires that we be guided by moral considerations. Health care ethics, also called medical ethics, biomedical ethics, and bioethics, is normative ethics specific to the health sciences: it raises the question of what is right or what ought to be done in a health science situation when a moral decision is called for. Such situations range from moral decisions in the clinical setting focused on one patient and his family to those concerned with policy decisions as to distribution of resources. Specifically, health care ethics addresses four interrelated areas: (1) clinical; (2) allocation of scarce resources; (3) human experimentation; and (4) health policy. It has been argued that moral considerations in the health sciences do not differ from normal, everyday moral considerations in that both work with the same moral principles and rules and use ethical reasoning. In health care ethics, the difference occurs only in the special situations and issues confronting the practitioner. The task of health care ethics therefore is neither to discover some new moral principles on which to build a theoretical ethical system nor to evolve new approaches to ethical reasoning, but to prepare the ground for the application of the established general moral principles and rules. In short, health care ethics is applied ethics. As with general ethics, we cannot expect an automatic deductive procedure in health care ethics for arriving at "the" ethical answer, nor can we legitimately expect ethics as a discipline to motivate those of us in the health sciences to be moral or to reprimand us when we are not. Health care ethics does not promote a particular moral life-style nor does it campaign for particular life values. Its role has been defined as functioning (1) to sensitize or raise the consciousness of health professionals (and the lay public) concerning ethical issues found in health care settings and policies; and (2) to structure the issues so that ethically relevant threads of complex situations can be drawn out. Health care ethics can illuminate the variety of conflicting ethical principles involved in a particular situation and can isolate pivotal concepts needing definition, clarification, or defense. Principles and theories taken from ethics and applied in the health care arena give us ways to systematically reason through an ethical dilemma.

HEALTH CARE ETHICS AND THE LAW

Law and ethics in a given society are similar in that they have developed in the same historical, social, cultural, and philosophical soil, but they also differ in some important ways. Smith and Davis indicated that it is possible to view the relationship between ethics and law as a four-way grid. Actions can be: (1) ethical and legal; (2) unethical and illegal; (3) ethical and illegal; and (4) unethical and legal. The latter two possibilities confront health professionals and present the most difficult situations to work through to some satisfactory solution.[13]

Because we use the term *right* in a very broad and indiscriminate way, the law can be helpful in giving us clues toward limiting this term to a workable definition and therefore to a more appropriate meaning. Legal rights are grounded in the law whereas ethical rights are grounded in ethical principles and rules. Positive rights mean that one has a right to something and negative rights mean that one has a right to be left alone. Free speech is a positive right, whereas refusing an injection is a negative right.

In health care ethics, situations involving rights and duties have at times reached the court. Two examples can illuminate the concepts of right and duty, as dealt with by the legal system. In the case *Canterbury v Spence*,[14] the patient underwent a laminectomy and within 24 hours after surgery fell while unattended and developed paralysis. The legal issues revolved around three factors: (1) informed consent; (2) negligence on the part of the physician performing the surgery; and (3) negligence on the part of the hospital in leaving the patient unattended while voiding immediately after the operation. To examine only the first factor, the concept of informed consent is based on the belief that an individual has the right to be informed regarding possible risks and benefits of a given procedure as well as alternatives to the procedure, including the alternative of no treatment, and their potential outcomes. Only by being fully informed can the patient truly consent to a procedure, since consent grounded in ignorance violates the individual's right to self-determination. One legal question in *Canterbury v Spence* focused on whether a 1 percent possibility of paralysis resulting from laminectomy, as documented in the literature, constituted peril of sufficient magnitude to bring a disclosure study into play. In other words, had the physician violated the patient's rights to know risks and benefits of the surgery by not performing his duty to disclose this information?

Another legal case, that of *Wyatt v Stickney*, dealt with the right to treatment.[15] Mr. Wyatt, like most of the patients at the state mental hospital in Alabama where Dr. Stickney functioned as Commissioner of Mental Health, had been involuntarily committed through noncriminal procedures. The lawyers argued that when patients are so committed for treatment purposes, they then unquestionably have a constitutional right to receive such individual treatment as will give each of them a realistic opportunity to be cured or to improve his or her mental condition. The argument continued that to deprive any citizen of his or her liberty upon the altruistic theory that the confinement is for humane, therapeutic reasons and then fail to provide adequate treatment violates the very fundamentals of due process. This case and the previously discussed one reflect the legal ramifications of ethical situations. Legislation and such documents as the Constitution with its Bill of Rights serve to connect the ethical concepts of a society with its legal system when ethical dilemmas must be solved in the courts. Legal and ethical questions continue to reach the courts and the newspapers and address an array of complex issues, such as the right to die, the right to treatment, whether one ought to donate an organ, the rights of defective newborns, reproductive technology, and legalized abortion. Recently, a married couple who had two children with a hereditary disorder decided they would not have more children. The husband had a vasectomy but the wife became pregnant after this surgery. This third child has neurofibromatosis and is retarded. The parents, on behalf of the child, sued their physician in a wrongful life or wrongful birth suit. The claim is that the child should not have been born but was so, and therefore damages are due from the physician for pain and suffering, the cost of treatment and care, and for loss of future earnings.[16]

ETHICAL DILEMMAS

As indicated earlier, one of the major difficulties in ethical discourses is that no definite, clear-cut answer exists for all ethical dilemmas. For that reason, critical reflection becomes necessary in any attempt to deal with an ethical dilemma. A dilemma can be defined as (1) a difficult problem seemingly incapable of a satisfactory solution; or (2) a situation involving choice between equally unsatisfactory alternatives. Not all dilemmas in life are ethical in nature, but an ethical dilemma does arise when moral claims conflict with one another. For example, we ought to prolong life and we ought to relieve suffering. Ethical dilemmas are situations involving conflicting moral claims, and give rise to such questions as: What ought I to do? What harm and benefit result from this decision or action? For example, in a situation where moral claims conflict, what one considers "good" may not necessarily be "right." This reveals a conflict between two moral claims, virtue and duty. Euthanasia may be considered good (a virtue) by some in a particular situation, but it may not be considered right (a duty). Another less dramatic example, but one that may occur more often, concerns the conflict between the patient's right to autonomy and the health professional's interference with and limitation of that right in the name of health. In this instance, the violation of patient autonomy by a decision to withhold information becomes justified because this is considered to be in the best interest of the patient. What is important to note here is that another is determining the best interest of the patient, rather than the patient himself making a decision after discussing the situation with appropriate health professionals. This behavior on the part of health professionals has been referred to by some as paternalism, where the health professional's behavior reduces the adult patient or the parents of the young patient to something less than decision-making, autonomous individuals.

Another example of conflicting moral claims arose in the case in which a hospital superintendent applied to the court for an order authorizing the administration of a blood transfusion. The court held that the adult patient had a right on religious grounds to refuse a blood transfusion, even if medical opinion was that the patient's decision not to accept blood amounted to the patient's taking his own life. The court determined that the patient had been mentally competent at all times when being presented with the decision that he had to make and was also competent when he made the decision. The court then concluded that the individual patient, the subject of a medical decision, must have the final say and that this must necessarily be so in a system of government that gives the greatest possible protection to the individual in the furtherance of his own desire.[17] The court in this case dealt with a conflict between the patient's right to refuse treatment and the doctor's duty to give treatment based on his medical judgment.

In the New York Hospital patient's bill of rights, one section, "Your Right to Decline Treatment," also addresses this ethical dilemma. It makes the point that patients do have the right to decline treatment but also says that if the hospital staff believes that a patient's decision to decline treatment is seriously inconsistent with its ability to provide the patient with adequate care, the patient may be requested to make arrangements elsewhere.[18] This clearly draws the ethical dilemma as a conflict between the patient's right to refuse treatment and the hospital staff's duty to provide treatment.

Yet another example of an ethical dilemma can be found in the clinical research situation. For the purposes of discussion, let us say that a clinical researcher has developed what appears to be an effective therapeutic technique and he wishes to test its efficacy among hospital patients who have the disease this technique is designed to cure. For comparative purposes, he divides the patients into two groups by random assignment so that the experimental group will receive the new technique and the control group will receive the currently accepted therapy. After a period of time elapses, the researcher discovers that one group seems to be recovering more rapidly than the other. Regardless of which group recovers faster, an ethical dilemma has been created by the conflict between, on the one hand, the obligation of the scientist to complete the experiment in order to add to knowledge that can help patients in the future and, on the other hand, the obligation of the clinician to provide the present patients with the most effective treatment available.[19] Other research situations call attention to different ethical dilemmas. Research involving children,[20] clinical research using a sample of elderly patients,[21] and research that uses a placebo[22] are only three examples of such situations.

The concept of health care as a right rather than a privilege has gained broad acceptance among many groups. In the arena of public policy, attempts continue to make this philosophical stance fit with the realities of health care delivery. The preamble to the World Health Organization Constitution says that the enjoyment of the highest attainable standard of health is one of the fundamental rights of every human being, without distinction on the basis of race, religion, political belief, or economic or social conditions.[23] In the United States at present, the vast majority of private health insurance plans are geared to the gainfully employed, with limited protection for the low-wage worker and none for the unemployed and the poor. The attempt to define health care as a right of citizen rather than as a commodity available according to the personal resources of the consumer has given us Medicare and Medicaid and has been the basis for the ongoing discussion regarding national health insurance. At present, access to health care is distributed inequitably, favoring the insured, the wealthy, and whites.[24]

With present economic problems and policies, health and social programs are in danger. The broader and ethical question here is: How does one account for societal callousness and indifference when they appear to coexist with a deep and abiding societal concern for others? Perhaps this conflict arises because in our world view we see society as operating in a consistent, just manner, so that the bad are punished and the good are rewarded. But is the world really this simple? Or perhaps the conflict can be explained by the observation that those who are doing well blame the victims, since to do so seems to relieve them of any felt obligation.

Discussion of any number of ethical dilemmas will occur not only during the development of public policy but will continue even after policy becomes enacted into law. The possibility of legislating ethical dilemmas out of the health care scene seems extremely remote. Regardless of the type of health care system, ethical dilemmas will continue to confront health care providers. A recent topic that has received much attention is that of rationing scarce medical resources. Numerous ethical questions arise, such as: Who should get what when not everyone can get what he or she needs to live? If medical resources are rationed, what criteria should be used to determine their allocation? Would such criteria as age, benefit to patient, contribution to society, and so forth be ethical?[25-27]

PROFESSIONAL OATHS AND CODES OF ETHICS IN THE HEALTH SCIENCES

Health care ethics, concerned as it is with rights, duties, and obligations, calls for an interdisciplinary quest for the structures of responsibility.[28] To understand the present situation, an examination of professional oaths and codes of ethics of the remote and recent past should prove fruitful. Although all health professional groups have oaths codes, this discussion focuses only on those of medicine and nursing.

Hippocrates, born on the island of Cos in the fifth century BC, became well known throughout Greece as a practicing physician. His attitude toward medicine threw off the religious aspects of suffering and made a beginning toward the scientific study of disease.[29] Today we remember him best for the Hippocratic Oath that doctors have traditionally taken upon graduation from medical school.

The Hippocratic Oath

I swear by Apollo Physician and Asclepius and Hygeia and Panakeia and all the gods and goddesses, making them my witnesses, that I will fulfill according to my ability and judgment this oath and this covenant:

To hold him who has taught me this art as equal to my parents and to live my life in partnership with him, and if he is in need of money to give him a share of mine, and to regard his offspring as equal to my brothers in male lineage and to teach them this art—if they desire to learn it—without fee and covenant; to give a share of precepts and oral instructions and all the other learning to my sons and to the sons of him who has instructed me and to pupils who have signed the covenant and have taken an oath according to the medical law, but to no one else.

I will apply dietetic measures for the benefit of the sick according to my ability and judgment; I will keep them from harm and injustice.

I will neither give a deadly drug to anybody if asked for it, nor will I make a suggestion to this effect. Similarly I will not give to a woman an abortive remedy. In purity and holiness I will guard my life and my art.

I will not use the knife, not even on sufferers from stone, but will withdraw in favor of such men as are engaged in this work.

Whatever houses I may visit, I will come for the benefit of the sick remaining free of all intentional injustice, of all mischief, and in particular of sexual relations with both female and male persons, be they free or slaves.

What I may see or hear in the course of the treatment or even outside of the treatment in regard to the life of men, which on no account one must spread abroad, I will keep to myself holding such things shameful [more accurately: 'unspeakable'] to be spoken about.

If I fulfill this oath and do not violate it, may it be granted to me to enjoy life and art, being honored with fame among all men for all time to come; if I transgress it and swear falsely, may the opposite of all this be true.

Primarily a pronouncement of medical ethics, this oath is not a set of laws enforced upon physicians by an authority but rather a guide which they accept of their own free will. Far from being a legal document, the Hippocratic Oath is a solemn promise given by the conscience of the physician who swears to it. The doctor's oath can be found in a number of variant forms, such as Christian, Arabic and Buddhist, and the Oath of Charaka used in India, and all share some similarities.

The Hippocratic tradition in medicine has led Paul Ramsey to remark that no profession comes close to medicine in its concern to inculcate, transmit, and keep in constant repair its standards governing the conduct of its members. The strengths of the Hippocratic tradition, a vital center of responsible medicine today, emphasize the importance of covenant fidelity between physician and student and physician and patient. Medicine functions, as a social contract, on the basis of this covenant. Again, Ramsey says that justice, fairness, righteousness, faithfulness, canons of loyalty, the sanctity of life, agape, or charity are some of the names given to the moral quality of attitudes and of action owed by any individual who steps into a covenant with another.[30] The Hippocratic tradition also reveals several weaknesses. Both the ethical and medical conceptions are pretechnological and thus there are limits in using them to probe the problems posed by technology. In addition, the tradition's focus on crisis treatment, as opposed to health promotion and maintenance and the model of the physician as a receptacle to whom people come require reexamination. Nevertheless, the oath has not only survived all these centuries but, because it anchors responsibility in the moral power and ability of the human being, it exerts influence on the practice of medicine today.

In 1971 the Judicial Council of the American Medical Association developed ethical principles to serve as standards of conduct for the physician. They address the duties, obligations, and rights of the medical practitioner. In 1980 these principles were revised, and reduced to seven, and now read as follows:

American Medical Association Principles of Medical Ethics

Preamble:
The medical profession has long subscribed to a body of ethical statements developed primarily for the benefit of the patient. As a member of this profession, a physician must recognize responsibility not only to patients, but also to society, to other health professionals, and to self. The following Principles adopted by the American Medical Association are not laws, but standards of conduct which define the essentials of honorable behavior for the physician.

I.
A physician shall be dedicated to providing competent medical service with compassion and respect for human dignity.

II.
A physician shall deal honestly with patients and colleagues, and strive to expose those physicians deficient in character or competence, or who engage in fraud or deception.

III.
A physician shall respect the law and also recognize a responsibility to seek changes in those requirements which are contrary to the best interests of the patient.

IV.

A physician shall respect the rights of patients, of colleagues, and of other health professionals, and shall safeguard patient confidences within the constraints of the law.

V.

A physician shall continue to study, apply and advance scientific knowledge, make relevant information available to patients, colleagues, and the public, obtain consultation, and use the talents of other health professionals when indicated.

VI.

A physician shall, in the provision of appropriate patient care, except in emergencies, be free to choose whom to serve, with whom to associate, and the environment in which to provide medical services.

VII.

A physician shall recognize a responsibility to participate in activities contributing to an improved community.*

In 1948 the general assembly of the World Medical Association in Geneva adopted an International Code of Medical Ethics and the Declaration of Geneva. These documents served to reaffirm the traditional professional commitments of the physician.

Before the late nineteenth century, nursing was closely allied with religion and religious orders, so its practitioners followed the ethics developed within these religious contexts. With the social change accompanying industrialization in England, nursing began to be practiced by untrained and socially marginal individuals. Florence Nightingale (1820–1910), the founder of modern nursing, became famous for her organizational and training endeavor for nurses during the Crimean War; later, in 1860, she opened the Nightingale Nursing School at St. Thomas's Hospital, London. In an 1893 paper, she wrote that sick persons must be treated rather than the disease, that prevention is infinitely better than cure, that universal hospitalization will not give positive health, and that nursing must hold to its ideals but must change some of its methods.[31] These ideals she referred to are reflected in a pledge that countless nurses around the world have taken.

The Florence Nightingale Pledge

I solemnly pledge myself before God and in presence of this assembly;

To pass my life in purity and to practice my profession faithfully;

Principles of Medical Ethics of the AMA, 1990. Reprinted with permission of the American Medical Association.

I will abstain from whatever is deleterious and mischievous and will not take or knowingly administer any harmful drug.

I will do all in my power to maintain and elevate the standard of my profession and will hold in confidence all personal matters committed to my keeping and family affairs coming to my knowledge in the practice of my calling.

With loyalty will endeavor to aid the physician in his work, and devote myself to the welfare of those committed to my care.

The International Council of Nurses in Geneva updated its code of ethics in 1973. This document addresses the duties, obligations, and rights that nurses have:

1973 Code for Nurses

Ethical Concepts Applied to Nursing
The fundamental responsibility of the nurse is fourfold: to promote health, to prevent illness, to restore health, and to alleviate suffering.

The need for nursing is universal. Inherent in nursing is respect for life, dignity, and rights of man. It is unrestricted by considerations of nationality, race, creed, color, age, sex, politics, or social status.

Nurses render health services to the individual, the family, and the community and coordinate their services with those of related groups.

Nurses and People
The nurse's primary responsibility is to those people who require nursing care.

The nurse, in providing care, respects the beliefs, values, and customs of the individual.

The nurse holds in confidence personal information and uses judgment in sharing this information.

Nurses and Practice
The nurse carries personal responsibility for nursing practice and for maintaining competence by continual learning.

The nurse maintains the highest standards of nursing care possible within the reality of a specific situation.

The nurse uses judgment in relation to individual competence when accepting and delegating responsibilities.

The nurse when acting in a professional capacity should at all times maintain standards of personal conduct that would reflect credit upon the profession.

Nurses and Society
The nurse shares with other citizens the responsibility for initiating and supporting action to meet the health and social needs of the public.

Nurses and Co-Workers
The nurse sustains a cooperative relationship with co-workers in nursing and other fields.

The nurse takes appropriate action to safeguard the individual when his care is endangered by a co-worker or any other person.

Nurses and the Profession
The nurse plays the major role in determining and implementing desirable standards of nursing practice and nursing education.

The nurse is active in developing a core of professional knowledge.

The nurse, acting through the professional organization, participates in establishing and maintaining equitable social and economic working conditions in nursing.*

In order to provide one means of professional self-regulation, the American Nurses' Association (ANA) revised its code of ethics, which had originally been adopted in 1950.[32] The Code for Nurses (1976) indicates the nursing profession's acceptance of the responsibility and trust with which it has been invested by society. The requirements of the Code may often exceed, but are not less than, those of the law. While violation of the law subjects the nurse to criminal or civil liability, the Association may reprimand, censure, suspend, or expel members from the Association for violation of the Code. The Interpretative Statement that accompanies the ANA Code outlines the ethical principles that underpin each section of the Code.

Code for Nurses

1. The nurse provides services with respect for human dignity and the uniqueness of the client unrestricted by considerations of social or economic status, personal attributes, or the nature of health problems.
2. The nurse safeguards the client's right to privacy by judiciously protecting information of a confidential nature.
3. The nurse acts to safeguard the client and the public when health care and safety are affected by the incompetent, unethical, or illegal practice of any person.
4. The nurse assumes responsibility and accountability for individual nursing judgments and actions.
5. The nurse maintains competence in nursing.
6. The nurse exercises informed judgment and uses individual competence and qualifications as criteria in seeking consultation, accepting responsibilities, and delegating nursing activities to others.
7. The nurse participates in activities that contribute to the ongoing development of the profession's body of knowledge.

---

*Reprinted with permission of the International Council of Nurses.

8. The nurse participates in the profession's efforts to implement and improve standards of nursing.
9. The nurse participates in the profession's efforts to establish and maintain conditions of employment conducive to high-quality nursing care.
10. The nurse participates in the profession's effort to protect the public from misinformation and misrepresentation and to maintain the integrity of nursing.
11. The nurse collaborates with members of the health professions and other citizens in promoting community and national efforts to meet the health needs of the public*

One tradition that evolved from historical events in this century must be included in any discussion of health care ethics. The ethos of the health sciences, particularly its experimental concepts, has been profoundly influenced by the Nuremberg experience. The Nazi medical experiments conducted during the Second World War had their genesis in a number of historical and social trends. In the 1800s, German medicine and universities participated in the insidious beginnings of twentieth century anti-Semitism. A number of changes affected the physician who, no longer an individual entrepreneur, became responsible for expressing the values of the prevailing social order. By the 1920s, emphasis on public health and preventive medicine focused on the desire to perfect the Nordic "species" by eliminating all impurities and defects.

The horrors of Nazi medical research included such experiments on concentration camp inmates as sterilization, placing inmates in pressure chambers and forcing them to endure high-altitude atmospheres until they died, tests on the effects of weightlessness and rapid fall, and freezing experiments in ice and snow. The K-technology, or the science of killing, led the Nazis to inject inmates with lethal doses of typhus and other pathogens and to experiment on them with gas, gangrene wounds, bone grafting, and direct injections of potassium and cyanide into the heart. The physicians dissected inmates alive to observe brain and heart action. And finally, at the height of sadism, the motivation for the macabre experiments was to collect different shapes of skulls and to retrieve human skin in order to make lampshades. The Nazi physicians' immolation of medical ethics on a massive scale proceeded unopposed by the German medical profession.[33] Out of this experience came the Nuremberg Code, which gives us valuable insights and directives to current research involving human subjects. One of this code's contributions is the precision with which it discusses the criterion of informed consent. The single most important ethical legacy of the Nuremberg experience is that it reminds us of the potential evil in human

---

*Reprinted with permission of the American Nurses' Association.

beings and serves to constantly refute the myth of inevitable progress.

Although not an ethical code per se, the American Hospital Association (AHA) has developed a Statement on a Patient's Bill of Rights, which has implications for health care ethics. The patient has the right:

1. To considerate and respectful care.
2. To obtain from the physician information regarding his diagnosis, treatment, and prognosis.
3. To give informed consent before the start of any procedure or treatment.
4. To refuse treatment to the extent permitted by law.
5. To privacy concerning his own medical care program.
6. To confidential communication and records.
7. To expect that the hospital will make a reasonable response to a patient's request for service.
8. To information regarding the relationship of his hospital to other health and educational institutions insofar as his care is concerned.
9. To refuse to participate in research projects.
10. To expect reasonable continuity of care.
11. To examine and question his bill.
12. To know the hospital rules and regulations that apply to patients' conduct.[34]

One critic of the AHA Patient's Bill of Rights calls it a well-intended, though timid, document and objects because he believes that it perpetuates the very paternalism that precipitated the abuses. He maintains that such a document creates the impression that the hospital is granting these rights to the patient. But since these rights were vested in the patient to begin with, the hospital has no power to grant these rights. He argues that the title seems both pretentious and deceptive, since if the rights have been violated they have been done so by the hospital and its staff. In effect, the document returns to the patient, with an air of largesse, some of the rights hospitals previously stole from him.[35]

Three other documents, which are not discussed here but that speak of the concepts of human rights and that have implications for health care ethics, are the World Medical Association Helsinki Declaration of 1964, the Preamble to the World Health Organization Constitution, and the United Nations International Covenant on Human Rights. Since so many factors influence health and illness, these documents, addressing the larger social, economic, cultural, civil, and political rights, provide a matrix for health care ethics.

THE ROLE OF THE ETHICIST

To the extent that we confront and attempt to deal with ethical dilemmas in health care by ethical reasoning, we are assuming the role of an ethicist. Although, these individuals may not be directly involved in the care of the patient, they can help by bringing their particular expertise to the situation. Such a person can help to structure the ethical issues involved in any ethical dilemma and provide another perspective, drawing not so much from a background in the health sciences but from philosophy and theology. Some health care centers now have an ethicist on the staff to assist the physicians, nurses, and others who ultimately must resolve specific ethical dilemmas and act on the decisions made.[36,37] Many more have ethics committees. These committees will be discussed in Chapter 5.

Although we have ethicists and ethics committees in health care settings, the fact remains that each person is a moral agent. To the extent that we develop moral sensitivity and systematic ways of reasoning through an ethical dilemma, we will do a better job at being a moral agent and a patient advocate. As nurses are even more affected by these situations in the future, they will need to recognize ethical dilemmas as such and will need to be able to reason through these dilemmas so that they can participate actively in the decisions on and possible resolution of these dilemmas. It is important to be able to take a reasoned ethical stance and to be able to articulate and ethically justify it. Righteous indignation may have its place, but a reasoned ethical stance may have more impact in the decision-making process.

REFERENCES

1. Frankena WK: *Ethics*. 2nd ed. Englewood Cliffs, NJ: Prentice-Hall; 1973: p 6.
2. Ibid, p 7.
3. Billica K: To care or not to care for noncompliant patients. *Focus Crit Care* 2:122–25, April 1989.
4. Dunaway P: Decisions to discontinue intensive therapy, influence factors and approaches to decision-making. *Intensive Care Nurs* 4:106–11, September 1988.
5. Haddad AM: The dilemma of keeping confidences. *AORN J* 1:159, 162–164, July 1989.
6. Schaeter S: Patient advocacy: An ethical dilemma? *Focus Crit Care* 3:191–192, June 1989.
7. Fowler MDM: Acquired immunodeficiency syndrome and refusal to provide care. *Heart Lung* 2:213–215, March 1988.
8. Bok S: Truth-telling and deception in medicine. Aaron Therman Memorial Lecture, Beth Israel Hospital. Boston, November 1976.
9. Frankena WK: *Ethics*, p 2.
10. Raatikainen R: Values and ethical principles in nursing. *J Ad Nurs* 2:92–96, February 1989.
11. Melden AI (ed): *Ethical Theories*, 2nd ed. Englewood Cliffs, NJ: Prentice-Hall; 1967: p 3.
12. Hudson WD: *Modern Moral Philosophy*. Garden City, NY: Doubleday; 1980: p 1.

13. Smith SA, Davis AJ: Ethical dilemmas: Conflicts among rights, duties, and obligations. *Am J Nurs* 80:1463–1466, 1980.
14. *Canterbury v Spence*, 464 F2d 772 (DC Cir 1972).
15. *Wyatt v Stickney*, 325 F Supp 781 (MD Al 1971).
16. Suing for being born. *Newsweek* 53, March 8, 1982.
17. *Erickson v Dilgard*, 252 NYS 2d 705 (1962).
18. The New York Hospital: Your Bill of Rights. New York, 1976.
19. Babbie ER: *Science and Morality in Medicine*. Berkeley: University of California Press; 1970: pp 16–17.
20. Everson-Bates S: Research involving children: Ethical concerns and dilemmas. *J Pediatr Health Care* 2:234–239, September–October 1988.
21. Bell JA, et al: Clinical research in the elderly: Ethical and methodological considerations. *Drug Intell Clin Pharm* 12:1002–1007, December 1987.
22. Desmarais M: The nurse's ethical guide to placebo giving. *Calif Nurse* 4:12, May 1988.
23. World Health Organization: Preamble to the Constitution of the World Health Organization. Geneva: WHO; July 1948.
24. Churchill L: *Rationing Health Care in America: Perceptions and Principles of Justice*. Notre Dame, IN: University of Notre Dame Press; 1987: p 13.
25. Daniels N: *Just Health Care*. Cambridge: Cambridge University Press; 1985.
26. Dolenc DA, Daugherty CJ: DRGs: The counter revolution in financing health care. *Hasting Cent Rep* 15:19–29, June 1985.
27. Callahan D: *Setting Limits: Medical Goals in an Aging Society*. New York: Simon & Schuster; 1987.
28. Vaux K: *Biomedical Ethics*. New York: Harper & Row; 1974: p xvi.
29. *Hippocrates: The Theory and Practice of Medicine*. New York: Philosophical Library; 1964.
30. Ramsey P: *The Patient as Person*. New Haven; Yale University Press; 1970: pp xii–xiii.
31. Bishop NJ, Goldie S: *A Bio-Bibliography of Florence Nightingale*. London: International Council of Nurses; 1962.
32. Viens DC: A history of nursing's code of ethics. *Nurs Outlook* 1:45–49, January–February 1989.
33. Lifton RJ: *The Nazi Doctors*. New York: Basic Books; 1986.
34. American Hospital Association: Patient's Bill of Rights. Chicago; 1970.
35. Gaylin W: The patient's bill of rights. *Sat Rev Sci*. March 1973: p 22.
36. Fowler MDM: The role of the clinical ethicist. *Heart Lung*. 3:318–319, May 1986.
37. Fletcher J, Quist N, Jonsen A, et al: *Ethics Consultation in Health Care*. Ann Arbor, MI: Health Administration Press; 1989.

CHAPTER **2**

Value Clarification and Moral Development

VALUE CLARIFICATION

Few things in life are value-free. Values are basic to a given way of life and serve to give direction to life. Our values are often similar to our breathing in that they are taken for granted. We do not go through life aware of the fact that we are breathing and therefore we do not think of our breathing. In the same manner, we do not always realize that we have a given set of values or that a decision is based on these values. We do not always examine our values but simply accept them and act on them. Again, as with breathing, we are more apt to think about our values when something goes wrong, because we then become more aware of them, just as we become more aware of our breathing when we experience difficulty. It has, however, been said that an unexamined life is not worth living.

Value clarification is a process that fosters the identification of significant values.[1] In this process we examine what we believe about the truth, beauty, or worth of any thought, object, or behavior. We make value judgments every day, ranging from trivial choices to those that affect our whole lives. Every individual has some sense of value, and there has never been a society that is devoid of a value system. In more traditional societies, values are embedded in habit, custom, and traditions. In societies in which rapid change occurs, values can become a source of controversy and conflict.

The word *axiology*, which comes from the Greek *axios*, meaning "worthy," has come to be used for the study of the general theory of value. Ethics, the study of values in human conduct, and aesthetics, the study of values in art, are subspecialties within the larger specialty of axiology.

One of the major issues in the study of values is whether value judgments express knowledge or feelings. Ordinarily we can distinguish between judgments of fact and judgments of value; however, it is difficult to separate them completely. For example, when we say that a Georgia O'Keeffe painting is beautiful, that honesty is good, and that spouse abuse is wrong, are we making assertions about things that are true or false or are we expressing preferences and making entreaties? The observable characteristics of things enter into our appraisals of values, so that if conditions change, our evaluation often changes too. In short, value judgments can be fact-dependent.[2]

Philosophers do not agree on the definition of the term *value*, but in general it is possible to say that value judgments are judgments of appraisal. Beyond the basic definition problem, however, other problems exist. For example, how are people to choose the values by which they are to live? Widespread agreement has been reached in the Western philosophical tradition about the existence of certain groups of values: aesthetic, economic, intellectual, moral, religious, scientific, and so on, but agreement has not been reached on the number, nature, interrelationship, or rank in a scale of values, or on the principles to be used in selecting them.

Certain principles are generally accepted in philosophical discussions on the selection of values.

1. Intrinsic values are preferred to extrinsic values. When something is intrinsically valuable, it is good in itself—that is, it is valued for its own sake and not for its capacity to lead to something else. Most things we use in our daily life have extrinsic value—that is, they are means to the attainment of other things. These two categories of values are not necessarily mutually exclusive. For example, knowledge is a good in itself but it is also a means to other good things, such as jobs.
2. Values that are productive and relatively permanent are preferred over those that are less productive and less permanent. Social, intellectual, aesthetic, and religious values tend to provide us with more permanent satisfaction than do material values.
3. We ought to select our values on the basis of self-chosen ends or ideals. The values we seek should be *our* values, consistent with each other and with the demands that life makes on us.
4. Of two positive values, the most positive ought to be selected, and conversely, when we are in a position when we must choose between two evils, we ought to choose the lesser one.[3]

Steele and Harmon made the point that values clarification is not a set of rules that interfere with conscientious decision-making but rather fosters the making of choices and facilitates decision making.[4] Values clarification is a dynamic process that fosters the individual's understanding of himself.

According to Simon and Clark, an important part of values clarification is the public affirmation of values that we cherish or praise and the act of standing up and being counted as an espouser of one's values.[5] This does not mean that we have the right to impose our values on others. As a profession, nursing embraces certain values, which are reflected in the Code for Nurses found in Chapter 1. Nursing has social responsibilities to society that have been articulated.[6,7] However, not everyone thinks that nursing's collective values are voiced sufficiently.[8] Within the profession, although certain basic values tend to cement us as a group, we as individual nurses vary in our ethical stances and action.[9-11]

The American Association of Colleges of Nursing undertook a national survey on preparing students as moral agents. The survey obtained data about ethical dilemmas that senior nursing students had encountered and their assessment of the adequacy of their ethics education.[12] In all the ethical dilemmas identified, questions of value underlie the dilemma. Values are operationalized during moral reasoning.[13]

One first step in dealing with the ethical dilemmas confronting us in nursing practice is to engage in values clarification. Another is to have some understanding of ethical principles and theories so as to reason through a dilemma in a systematic way and be able to articulate a reasoned stance.

MORAL DEVELOPMENT

We have moved into the area called *moral development* when we raise such questions as: How does a person become moral? What do we mean when we say someone is a person of principle? What factors influence the way we behave in a moral situation? Moral development has been examined and studied from a variety of perspectives: cognitive–developmental psychology, psychoanalysis, psychobiology, social learning theory, social psychology, education, clinical psychology, political psychology, and social ecology. It is concerned with a vast range of theoretical and empirical issues in child development, adult behavior, violence, altruism, criminality, cooperation, honesty, child rearing, self-control, situational variations in behavior, modeling, social and political attitudes, personality functioning, and the impact of culture on socialization, to list some major foci in the area of moral development.

Kohlberg has evolved a cognitive–developmental theory of moral development. His theory has three levels of development: (1) preconventional morality; (2) conventional morality; and (3) postconventional or principled morality. Most children under 9 years of age and some adolescent and adult criminal offenders have limited moral development and are at the preconventional level. People at the conventional level of development tend to conform to and uphold the rules, expectations, and conventions of society or authority. Most adults and adolescents are at this level, according to Kohlberg. The postconventional level is reached by a minority of adults, usually only after the age of 20. These people have differentiated themselves from the rules and expectations of others and define their values in terms of self-chosen principles.[14-18]

In Kohlberg's theory, there is a parallel between an individual's logical or cognitive stage and that person's moral stage. While logical development is a necessary condition for moral development, it is not in itself sufficient, since many individuals are at a higher logical stage than the parallel moral stage. In addition, one can reason in terms of ethical principles if one is at the postconventional level and still not live up to them. A variety of factors determines whether a particular person will live up to his stage of moral reasoning and development. The individual's sense of justice is what is most distinctively and fundamentally moral. One can act morally and question all rules, and one can act morally and question the greater good, but one cannot act morally and question the need for justice.

Students of human development have faced a difficult problem when examining cultural variations in moral judgment. Values found across time and space are remarkably complex and diverse. The substance of morality—or the actual rules of ethical conduct, the values and mores that govern behavior—is deeply embedded in specific cultural patterns. When these scholars probe deeper and examine an abstract principle, such as justice, however, they find a more consistent pattern emerging. The structural function of values, or how a culture thinks about these principles, tends to be more stable than their content, or how the culture puts these principles into operation. Thus, values can be analyzed in terms of their common functional purposes and can be viewed as equivalents despite gross differences in specific content. Work done by Piaget and later by Kohlberg does not lend itself easily to the study of cultural variation, since these authors placed emphasis on essentially acultural invariant sequences. Others interested in the field of moral development have attempted to overcome this limitation and have developed a conception of moral development using a nonhierarchical typology.

An important question for us to consider is what factors influence the way we behave in a moral situation. Although it is sometimes difficult for us to come to grips with the notion that we are creatures of our environment, the difficulty increases when we examine the idea that some moral behavior is situationally determined. This is due in part to the fact that our conception of human responsibility is largely based on the assumption that the individual is responsible for his behavior. Nevertheless, analysis of the literature to determine whether morality is more strongly influenced by personality (beliefs, values, attitudes, etc.)

than by situations has led several writers to conclude that the latter are far more powerful influences.[19-21]

Nowhere are the data supporting the importance of situational determinants of moral behavior more compelling than in the reality of and research in the capacity of people to inflict great harm on others. Milgram's classic experiments on obedience provide an excellent example with which to illustrate this point. Milgram conducted research on obedience and in the name of science had his study sample of students "shock" learners with increasing voltages, including one setting marked "severe shock."[22] The results of these experiments do not fit our expectations. That is, we do not expect so many people to obey the experimenter and deliver such harsh pain. Research in this area generally does not point to a relationship between personality variables and behavioral obedience; rather, it seems that the tendency to be critical-minded and the possession of a high cognitive energy is related to the capacity to defy authority and to disobey.

The cumulative impact of these studies suggests that we are not the captains of our moral ships that we believe ourselves to be. Optimism comes from the fact that this research does suggest that situational factors can be arranged to maximize moral and prosocial behavior. It is conceivable that in a society or institution where situational support for prosocial behavior is strongly and consistently provided, many more people will develop the kind of moral system that no longer requires external supports.

CARING

In the past several years, there has been a growing body of literature that has posed a challenge to both traditional and contemporary assumptions underlying moral theory. The thesis in this new literature is that women undergo a moral development that is distinct from but parallel to that of men. The first to write on this idea that gender is an important variable in our moral life was Carol Gilligan, who studied with Kohlberg. In her book she distinguishes a morality of rights and formal reasoning, which she calls the justice perspective, from a morality of care and responsibility, or the care perspective. In the justice perspective, an autonomous moral agent discovers and applies a set of fundamental rules through the use of universal and abstract reason. In the care perspective, the central preoccupation is a responsiveness to others that dictates providing care, preventing harm, and maintaining relationships.[23] Gilligan also constructed a model of moral development but one that differs from Kohlberg's model. At the preconventional level, the orientation is toward individual survival. At the conventional level, the focus is on care and conformity and there is a concomitant desire to please others. At the postconventional level, care becomes a self-chosen principle, one that recognizes the interdependence of self and other. The individual has developed an increasing understanding of human relationships. As a self-in-relation, one attempts to maintain one's own integrity and care for one's self without neglecting others.

Within the context of feminist research and writings, Gilligan has reconceptualized women's moral perspective. Other writers have added to this literature.[24-28]

A number of nurses have also written about the importance of caring including Benner and Wrubel,[29] Carper,[30] and Watson.[31] This is a rich literature that addresses both the gender aspects of ethical reasoning and a core value of nursing. The nursing ethics literature has been examined and classified into three categories: (1) the application of the major consequential and deontological theories to ethical issues; (2) the use of traditional moral principles and ideals to guide discussion of moral problems; and (3) the philosophical foundations approach, in which ethical issues are dealt with from the perspective of a philosophical conception of the nature of nursing.[32] The caring principle is the bedrock of this third category.

Along with this more recent and important demonstration of the justice perspective and the care perspective, we also have the very ancient notion of virtues, or those qualities of character that make us a good person. Two basic questions confront us as moral agents: (1) what sort of person ought I to be? and (2) what ought I do in a given situation of conflicting moral claims? The first question addresses the question of what virtues one ought to have. The second question addresses the question of how one ethically reasons through an ethical dilemma when confronted with one.[33]

It is important to realize that justice or caring and virtues or reasoning are different concepts, and are not completely and mutually exclusive categories. Fowler has shown that ethics and virtues are interrelated.[34] Gilligan, while pointing to gender differences in moral development, also makes the point that women use both the justice perspective and the care perspective.

VALUE CLARIFICATION AND NURSING

It is important for nurses to examine their values and to clarify them. This can best occur in those situations in which we are honest with ourselves. We all have an idea of our selves, referred to as our self-concept. This includes our idealized selves and the values that we think we have and the ones that we really have. In addition, and importantly, there can be a discrepancy between what we value and what we do when these values are called into action.

In the past, socialization into nursing has often dealt with these questions of value by attempting to inject "proper" values into students. There was little, if any, examination of the complexity of values or of the failure to act on one's higher or idealized values. We believe that moral conflict or ethical dilemmas can provide nurses with moments in which they can grow both as moral individuals and as members of the nursing profession.

MORAL DEVELOPMENT AND NURSING

A number of studies of nurses and moral development have been reported in the literature. Murphy indicated that for nurses to function optimally in complex settings and to act as responsible moral agents, they need to attain a postconventional level of moral development. She went on to say that the collective morality prevalent in nursing has led to loss of personal integrity among nurses and has led them to more often blame others than to accept responsibility.[35]

Ketefian conducted a study with a sample of 79 practicing nurses, examining critical thinking, educational preparation, and development of moral judgment. She found that the higher the nurses' critical thinking, the higher they scored on moral reasoning. Nurses who had professional education had more advanced levels of moral reasoning than those who had received technical nursing preparation.[36] In addition to this first study, Ketefian has conducted three other important projects along this same line.[37-39]

Another study, measuring moral judgment and nursing dilemmas on the basis of the cognitive theory of moral development, investigated the difference between nurses' responses to general, hypothetical moral dilemmas and their responses to real-life nursing dilemmas. Findings verified the significance of formal education and previous involvement with similar dilemmas in enhancing principled thinking. This study also raises some questions about situational pressures, conflicting claims, and contexts of professional dilemmas.[40]

Such research, focused on nurses and moral development and moral judgment, is only in its initial stages. But already these studies provide us with food for thought and the basis for continued research. Two authors who have applied Gilligan's work to nursing maintain that if an ethical base for nursing practice is built on the ethics of justice and the nurse's orientation is the ethics of care, there will continue to be a denial of the nurse's own voice.[41]

These different voices, both from outside the nursing profession and from within it, point to the fact that the moral foundation of nursing will have to derive from bold excursions into the meaning of nursing.[42] And as one writer has said, nursing theory and nursing ethics are the two main areas of inquiry in nursing scholarship today. Both address similar theses and speak not only about but also for nursing. More dialogue between these two areas would provide us with a richer understanding of the nature of nursing.[43]

REFERENCES

1. Steele SM, Harmon VM: *Values Clarification in Nursing.* New York: Appleton-Century-Crofts; 1979: p 1.
2. Frisch NC: Value analysis. *J Nurs Educ* 26:328–332, 1987.
3. Fry ST: Teaching ethics in nursing curricula. *Nurs Clin North Am* 24:485–497, 1989.
4. Steele, Harmon VM: *Values*, p 7.
5. Simon SB, Clark J: *Beginning Values Clarification.* San Diego: Pennant; 1975.
6. American Nurses' Association: Nursing: A Social Policy Statement. Kansas City, MO: American Nurses' Association, 1980.
7. Davis AJ: Nursing as a socially responsible profession. Keynote address. Western Society for Research in Nursing Conference. Salt Lake City, UT; May 5, 1988.
8. Flanagin A: The ethical voice of nursing—I can't hear it, can you? *JOGN Nurs* 3:162–163, May–June 1988.
9. Hilbert GA: Moral development and unethical behavior among nursing students. *J Prof Nurs* 3:167–169, May–June 1988.
10. Ketefian S: A case study of theory development: Moral development in nursing. *ANS* 9:10–19, January, 1987.
11. Farrell B: AIDS patients: Values in conflict. *Crit Care Nurs Q* 10:74–85, September, 1987.
12. American Association of Colleges of Nursing: Special Report: RN Baccalaureate Nursing Education (1986–1989). Washington DC; The American Association of Colleges of Nursing and ASHE/ERIC (HED21745), 1989.
13. Omery A: Values, moral reasoning and ethics. *Nurs Clin North Am* 24:499–508, June, 1989.
14. Kohlberg L: Stage and sequence: The cognitive–developmental approach to socialization. In Goslin DA (ed): *Handbook of Socialization Theory and Research.* Chicago: Rand McNally; 1969: pp 347–480.
15. Kohlberg L, Kramer RB: Continuities and discontinuities in childhood and adult moral development. *Hum Dev* 12:93-120, 1969.
16. Kohlberg L: From is to ought. In Mischel T (ed): *Cognitive Development and Epistemology.* New York: Academic Press; 1971: pp 151–235.
17. Kohlberg L, Gilligan CF: The adolescent as philosopher: The discovery of the self in a postconventional world. *Daedalus* 100:1051–1086, 1971.
18. Kohlberg L: *The Philosophy of Moral Development.* New York: Harper & Row; 1981.
19. Moore BS, Underwood B, Rosenhan DL: Affect and Altruism. *Dev Psychol* 8:99–104, 1973.
20. Rosenhan DL, Underwood B, Moore BS: Affect moderates self-gratification and altruism. *J Pers Soc Psychol* 30:546–552, 1974.

21. Rosenhan DL, Moore BS, Underwood B: The social psychology of moral behavior. In Lickona T (ed): *Moral Development and Behavior.* New York: Holt, Rinehart & Winston; 1976.
22. Milgram S: Behavioral study of obedience. *J Abnorm Soc Psychol* 67:371–378, 1963.
23. Gillian C: *In a Different Voice.* Cambridge, MA: Harvard University Press; 1982.
24. McMillan C: *Women, Reason and Nature.* Princeton, NJ: Princeton University Press; 1982.
25. Chodrow N: *The Reproduction of Mothering.* Berkeley: University of California Press; 1978.
26. Miller JB: *Toward a New Psychology of Women.* Boston: Beacon Press; 1976.
27. Rich A: Of Woman Born. New York: Bantam Books; 1976.
28. Nodding N: Caring. Berkeley: University of California Press; 1984.
29. Benner P, Wrubel J: *The Primacy of Caring.* Menlo Park, CA: Addison-Wesley; 1989.
30. Carper BA: The ethics of caring. *ANS* 3:11–19, March 1979.
31. Watson J: Nursing: *The Philosophy and Science of Caring.* Boston: Little Brown; 1979.
32. Pence T: Approaches to nursing ethics. *Philos Context* 17:7–16, 1987.
33. Davis AJ: An international perspective on nursing ethics: Ethical relativism and ethical absolutes. Paper presented at the International Congress of Nurses, Seoul, Korea, June, 1989.
34. Fowler MDM: Ethics without virtue. *Heart Lung* 15:528–530, September, 1986.
35. Murphy CP: Models of the nurse–patient relationship. In Murphy C, Hunter H (eds): *Ethical Problems in the Nurse–Patient Relationship.* Boston Allyn & Bacon; 1983: pp 9–24.
36. Ketefian S: Critical thinking and educational preparation, and development of moral judgment among selected groups of practicing nurses. *Nurs Res* 30:98–103, March–April, 1981.
37. Ketefian S: Tool development in nursing: Construction of a scale to measure moral behavior. *J NY State Nurs Assoc* 13:13–18, 1982.
38. Ketefian S: Professional and bureaucratic role conceptions and moral behavior among nurses. *Nurs Res* 34:248–253, July–August, 1985.
39. Ketefian S: A case study of theory development: Moral behavior in nursing. *ANS* 9:2, 10–19, September, 1987.
40. Crisham P: Measuring moral judgment in nursing dilemmas. *Nurs Res* 30:104–110, March–April, 1981.
41. Huggins EA, Scalzi CC: Limitations and alternatives: Ethical practice theory in nursing. *ANS* 10:4, 43–47, October, 1988.
42. Packard JS, Ferrara MSN: In search of the moral foundation of nursing. *ANS* 10:4, 60–71, October, 1988.
43. Yeo M: Integration of nursing theory and nursing ethics. *ANS* 11:3, 33–42, April, 1989.

Selected Ethical Approaches

Ethical problems in the nursing profession are nothing new. Yet the development of new technologies and cost-containment efforts affect the nature and substance of these dilemmas in the interrelationships of nurses, patients, and physicians as individuals and as members of an increasingly complex society. Enlarged responsibilities for all health professionals are the outcomes in terms of decision making. Similar burdens also fall on consumers of health care.

The nurse as a moral agent is concerned with values, choices, priorities, and duties related to the "good" of the individual, the nursing profession, and the society. What is needed is a more systematic way of approaching ethical issues facing nursing at all levels, from the individual provider–patient encounter to the level of policy making for delivery of health and nursing care. The notion of an ethical approach suggests a reasoned process or ways of analyzing or conceptualizing decisions and choices in the ethical dimensions of practice rather than a reliance on ready-made answers or decisions based only on gut-level feelings. This chapter is a brief overview of selected historical and contemporary moral positions that can be considered in reflecting on those nurse–patient situations where the right decision is unclear and there are conflicts of rights and duties. These selected theories and positions of historical and contemporary ethicists may be used in clarifying the ethical dimensions of dilemmas in health care. The most commonly discussed positions in health care today are utilitarianism, often used in justifying resource allocation, and the deontological approach. While they do not provide answers per se, they do go beyond what Callahan called ethical slogans, or one-sentence general principles for justifying moral judgments and actions.[1] Articulation of opposing positions of decision makers brings into the open additional sources of conflict that need to be clarified in order to develop a responsible decision.

The general concern of ethics has to do with examining the moral basis for our judgments and actions, our duties and obligations. Moral philosophers, beginning with Socrates, Plato, and Aristotle, have for centuries attempted to answer two major questions of ethics: What is the meaning of right and of good? What is the morally right thing to do in this situation? The first question is in the area of metaethics; the second is in the area of normative or applied ethics. Health professionals are primarily concerned with the second question, concerning normative ethics. Normative ethics attempts to justify one form of behavior over another, to determine the right-making characteristics of action, for purposes of carrying out duties and obligations. The nurse, often in a situation vis-à-vis a patient, group, or community that requires the identification of alternative courses of action, must make a choice as to what he or she will do when there is a conflict of rights and obligations between patients, families, other health workers, or the community. Selected ethical theories will be discussed briefly to suggest how and what to consider in dealing with conflicts that require choices for action or nonaction in patient–provider relationships and in policy making.

One needs data to proceed with discussion of the question about the morally right thing to do in a given situation. The process of reflective thinking provides data by asking questions related to identifying the individuals involved in the situation, the required action(s), possible and probable consequences of the proposed action(s), the intention or purpose of the action(s), the range of alternatives or choices, and the context of the action(s). This process indicates that the methods of thinking in science and ethics are not mutually exclusive. One goes through a similar process in asking questions about the world of nature, on the one hand, and the world of ethics and values, on the other hand. The data base is different as are the variables considered. Both are systematic processes.

Various ethical positions provide different ways of structuring these data, which may lead to the same or different decisions for action. These approaches assume that the nurse has already identified a situation in which conflict of duties, obligations, or interests exists. The nurse seeks the "best" or "right" action to take when the alternatives seem equally undesirable—for example, lying versus truth telling, or allocation of scarce nursing manpower resources when nursing care is supposed to be based on need, one idea of distributive justice.

Because these dilemmas are frustrating and difficult to deal with it is essential that a spirit of compassion, caring, and community permeate discussion of them at all levels. There are no ready-made solutions to be found in books or in the laboratory.

TWO TRADITIONAL POSITIONS

The traditional positions or theories of deontology (formalism) and utilitarianism provide us with ways of looking at health care dilemmas from an ethical standpoint.

Deontology

The deontological or formalist ethical approach focuses on duties and suggests that the rightness or wrongness of actions depends on more than the nurse's pleasure or the consequences of the proposed action. Rightness or wrongness depends on the nature or form of these actions in terms of their inherent moral significance—e.g., keeping a promise. Moral significance is attached to certain relationships, as well. For example, the parent–child or the nurse–patient relationship establishes a basis for considering one's special duties and obligations. In this tradition, there are both act-deontologists and rule-deontologists—that is, obligations in relationships may be based on performing certain actions or adhering to certain rules or principles.

In act-deontology, the moral values of the individual nurse are of major significance. For example, in a given situation in the home setting, the moral values of the community health nurse would play an important part in decisions made about kinds of information given to the family. This position requires commitment to the principle of universalizability. That is, when one makes a moral judgment in one given situation, one will make the same judgment in any similar situation regardless of time, place, or persons involved. If one judges X to be right or good in this situation, then one must judge that anything like X is right or good in any similar situation.[2] In any home setting, given a similar situation, the nurse would give the same kinds of information— for example, on birth control methods. According to this theory, one has only rules of thumb to go by. There are no criteria, standards, or guiding principles to go by, as in rule-deontology. One simply gets all the facts and makes a decision. An act is made right simply by choosing it and by the agent's commitment to universalizing it.

Critics of act-deontology claim that it is not helpful in terms of moral guidance, because it is difficult to do without rules. One may not always have the time and energy to carefully judge each situation in and of itself.[3]

The rule-deontologist suggests that there are standards for choosing, judging and reasoning morally. The standard consists of fairly specific rules, such as keeping promises and never telling lies. These rules say that we should act in a certain way in a given situation. X is the right act because one should always tell the truth or do unto others as one would have others do to oneself—the golden rule.

One problem with rule-deontology is that rules sometimes conflict and one has to decide which rule takes precedence over another. Another problem is the exception to the rule. In dealing with this problem, Ross distinguished between actual duty and prima facie duty. He said that every rule of actual duty has exceptions, but prima facie duties have no exceptions. They are obligations that one must always try to fulfill—for example, fidelity, gratitude, and justice.[4] But what if prima facie duties conflict with each other in a given situation? For example, if a nurse is spending most of her time caring for a seriously ill patient, she cannot give her attention to other patients on her unit. While caring faithfully for one patient, the nurse may not be providing fair treatment to other patients on the unit.

A rule-deontologist might deal with conflict of prima facie duties by an appeal to the Divine Command Theory: an act is right or wrong because it is commanded or forbidden by God. This has problems for both believers and nonbelievers. If God commands cruelty and injustice, then it is obligatory to carry out a cruel or unjust act, a dilemma for a moral agent.[5]

Immanuel Kant provided another possible way out of the problem of conflicting rules. Writing in the late eighteenth century, he stated that one should "act only on that maxim which you can at the same time will to be a universal law," the major form of the categorical imperative.[6] An example of this imperative is a nurse asking another nurse, "What if everyone did what you're doing?" when the first nurse sees the second nurse taking patient medications for her own use. Another form of the categorical imperative says that persons should always be treated as ends and never as means. This can be a problem for a nurse researcher who uses human subjects primarily as means to a particular research goal.

Kant said that categorical imperatives are unconditional commands, morally necessary and obligatory under any circumstances.[7] It is one's duty to obey categorical imperatives, with no exceptions. One does not look at the consequences. There is no external authority to tell one what to do.[8]

Kant's approach does not help us with the resolution of specific moral conflicts. When one tries to apply the Kantian approach, it is difficult to separate the idea of duty and obligations from ends, purposes, wants, and needs in a given situation. For example, if the goal is to return the institutionalized mentally retarded to the community, what happens to the specific needs of a mentally retarded adult who may not be able to live outside an institution and has no family? What is the health provider's obligation?

In summary, the deontological position focuses on the moral significance of the values of the agent and on duties and obligations guided by specific rules and principles without regard to consequences. This position does not help the agent resolve a situation in which duties and obligations conflict. It does not resolve the dilemma for the nurse who decides to follow the rule that one should always tell the truth but realizes that the truth will undoubtedly hurt a particular patient in a given situation where the principle of telling the truth conflicts with the principle of doing no harm.

Utilitarianism

The theory of utility focuses on consequences of decisions and actions, and defines *good* as happiness or pleasure and *right* as maximizing the greatest good and least amount of harm for the greatest number of persons. This position assumes that one can weigh and measure harm and benefit and come out with the greatest possible balance of good over evil for most people.

Bentham and Mill have presented the major historical arguments for the position of utility as a standard against which the rightness and wrongness of actions are to be compared. This position, sometimes known as "calculus morality," calculates the effects of all alternative actions on the general welfare of present and future generations in a given situation. Some moral philosophers distinguish between rule- and act-utilitarianism. One seeks to determine acts and rules having the greatest utility in a broad sense of usefulness, pleasure, and happiness. The agent looks at actions and rules in terms of what the consequences would be for the general welfare if everyone acted similarly in a given situation.[9] What if every hospital decided to perform liver and heart transplants and to close the emergency room? What would be the consequences for the population that needs primary care services?

One is immediately faced with the problem of whether this position involves the total happiness for a few or the average happiness for all. A crucial question is whether or not what one does in a particular situation contributes to the greatest general good or the least amount of harm for everyone. But how can everyone's welfare really be considered? Critics bring up several other problems. They accuse the utilitarian of ignoring the personal nature of good—for example, in truth telling and promise keeping. All actions need not be considered in light of the overall general welfare. Individuals do count. The utilitarian tradition is often invoked in making decisions about the funding of health care. This is in direct conflict with the medical ethic, whereby one does everything possible for the individual patient. Certain groups may accept benefits without making any sacrifices, raising the question of justice and fairness. Utility is not the only criterion in making moral judgments. Actually, if one adds the notion of distributing the good as widely as possible through society, one adds the principle of justice to the principle of utility for making ethical judgments. This is no longer pure utilitarianism. From this point of view, utility by itself cannot be the only basic standard or first principle of right and wrong.[10]

To summarize, deontological and utilitarian traditions offer different perspectives from which moral judgments might be made. Each position has strengths and limitations when applied to specific ethical dilemmas in nursing and health care delivery.

CONTEMPORARY POSITIONS

Some modern philosophers offer other positions from which to look at ethical dilemmas and get beyond the unresolved problems one is left with in the deontological and utilitarian traditions. Shades of utilitarian and deontological thinking may be detected in some of these newer positions.

Theory of Obligation

Frankena's theory of obligation considers two principles as basic: the principle of beneficence and the principle of justice as equal treatment. The principle of beneficence asks us not just to want the good but to actually do good and not evil. According to Frankena, the principle of beneficence has four "oughts": (1) not to inflict harm or evil; (2) to prevent harm; (3) to remove evil; and (4) to do or promote good.[11] This theory has more in common with the deontological tradition.

The principle of justice or distributive justice is the equal or comparative treatment of individuals. Distributive justice seeks to distribute benefits and burdens equally throughout society. Criteria suggested as a basis for the exercise of distributive justice are: (1) dealing with people according to their merits; (2) treating people as equals in distributing good and evil equally among everyone; and (3) treating people according to their needs.[12] In our society, there is no consensus as to what criterion will be used in seeking the most just way of distributing goods, such as health care. A criterion that is invoked more frequently with cost-containment efforts is the ability to pay. The nursing literature, such as the American Nurses' Association (ANA) Code for Nurses, addresses care based on need, which is only one way of ordering priorities and distributing nursing and health care.

These two principles of justice and beneficence may come into conflict at the individual action level and at the policy-making level. Additional dimensions of the principles are included in the next chapter. Frankena suggested that as we approximate solutions to ethical dilemmas in a cooperative effort at a given point in time, these two principles will not be inconsistent. An example of trying to apply these principles at the policy level is the work of the interdisciplinary President's Commission for the Study of Ethical Problems in Medicine and Biomedical and Behavioral Research as it dealt with access to health care.

The Ideal Observer Theory

Firth proposed the "ideal observer" theory as an approach to making moral judgments. This is a theory of cognitive processes and characteristics. The qualities of consistency, disinterestedness, dispassionateness, omniprecipience, omniscience, and normality characterize the "ideal observer" or moral judge, which could be an individual or a machine—for example, a computer. Omniscience means obtaining all the information one can about the situation in question. No limits are put on what the "ideal observer" should know. No information can be censored. Omniprecipience, a word coined by Firth, is the ability to see implications and consequences of projected actions as if one were experiencing them. One uses all one's powers of imagination to do this, with the awareness that one can never totally enter into another person's experience. Some would call this empathy.[13]

Dispassionateness and disinterestedness refer to impartiality. One is impartial in the sense that one has no special interests or relationships to the given dilemma. The "ideal observer" has only general interests, such as the welfare of all, and does not experience jealousy or any similar emotions directed to particular individuals. To experience such emotions is to be disqualified as a moral judge. Impartiality also assumes equal treatment for everyone in similar situations.[14]

The notion of consistency refers to ethical decisions made in two different situations. These decisions must be consistent with each other in the sense that any "ideal observer" would react in the same manner to a given set of circumstances even though they might vary with the culture. Consistency follows from the other qualities discussed in combination with recognized laws of psychological behavior. In other respects, the "ideal observer" falls within the range of "normality."[15] He or she observes the physical and mental conditions favorable for making valid decisions—that is, he or she is not sick, hungry, cold, tired, or suffering from jet lag.

This theory provides us with characteristics of ethical reasoning and reflective thinking processes and provides us with some criteria for examining ethical dilemmas and alternatives for action from the point of view of an "ideal observer." It also provides some assistance to health professionals in deciding when they should *not* be the judge in a given situation and should seek the help of disinterested others, such as an ethics committee or the courts, when patients or clients are unable to make their own decisions.

Justice as Fairness

Rawls discusses justice as fairness and as the foundation of social structures. Justice, broadly speaking, has to do with the distribution of good and evil, harms and benefits in society. According to Rawls, the principles of justice have to do with distribution of what he called primary goods: income, wealth, liberty, opportunity, and the bases of self-respect. His theory offers us another perspective from which to view ethical decision making and the basis for moral decisions. It is a rethinking of the social contract theory of obligation in the Kantian tradition. The heart of the theory is the notion of the "original position" in which people come together to negotiate the principles of justice by which all are bound to live. The negotiators are rational, intelligent people who wish to pursue their own life plans in a more just society.[16]

Rawls placed the negotiators under the constraints of a "veil of ignorance" They have knowledge and facts about such general fields as sociology and economics. They do not know any particular facts about themselves or others—for example, personal characteristics, sex, social class. The purpose of the "veil of ignorance" is to remove from the negotiations any possibility of individuals seeking to satisfy their own interests at the expense of others. This is the situation referred to as the "original position." The negotiators must favor only those principles that advance everyone's best interests. The employee might turn out to be of the least fortunate individuals in a given community.[17] In the end, the negotiators must arrive at what Rawls called "justice as fairness," because they do negotiate behind the "veil of ignorance" to form the basic principles of society.

The concept of "justice as fairness" is articulated in two basic principles of justice: (1) each person is to have an equal right to the most extensive system of liberty for all; and (2) social and economic inequalities are to be arranged so that they are to the greatest benefit of the least fortunate and are attached to offices and positions open to everyone under conditions of equality of opportunity.[18] The first principle, maximizing liberty for all, has absolute priority over the second if and when the two principles conflict.

Rawls also discussed five criteria for looking at the rightness of any ethical principles: (1) universality (i.e., the same principles must hold for everyone in similar situations); (2) generality (i.e., the principles must not refer to specific people or situations, such as my mother or your marriage); (3) publicity (i.e., they must be known and recognized by all involved); (4) ordering (i.e., they must somehow order conflicting claims without resort to force); and (5) finality (i.e., they may override the demands of law and custom).[19] Nurses could use these criteria to look at their own moral principles and values, those proposed by other health professionals, or those assumed in a policy for health care delivery to those who are uninsured.

In considering "justice as fairness," inequalities are allowed only to improve the condition of the least fortunate—for example, children, the elderly, the poor. The least advantaged are in the normative position in society. Basic rights and obligations proceed from the notion of fairness for these disadvantaged groups. Vaux said that this is invoking the golden rule in such a way that one is truly committed to the well-being of another.[20] Justice as fairness to the least advantaged becomes the categorical imperative in the Kantian tradition.

Rawls made no claim that his theory could be applied directly in contemporary society. However, he has provided us with a new way to look at moral problems in society generally and specifically in health care. Other philosophers are considering the implications of Rawls' ideas for development of a more just health care system (see Chapter 4). How might the health care system look if the least fortunate were considered first in a public policy decision on allocation of health manpower resources or funding for health care programs?

The contemporary ethical positions discussed here can be accepted or rejected on a variety of grounds as plausible ways of looking at ethical dilemmas in health care. The following is a summary of the ethical positions discussed:

SUMMARY OF SELECTED ETHICAL
THEORIES OR APPROACHES

Theory or Approach	What Makes a Decision or Action "Right"
1. Deontology or formalism	The moral agent should consider the inherent nature of an act or rule rather than the consequences—for example, one should never tell a lie. Focus is on duties and obligations.
2. Utilitarianism	The moral agent should consider consequences of rules and acts and seek the greatest possible balance of happiness over unhappiness for the greatest number. This implies that good and evil can be measured and balanced in some way.
3. Obligation: beneficence and justice (Frankena)	The moral agent should consider rules and actions from a basis of the principles of beneficence and justice as equality.
4. Ideal observer (Firth)	The moral agent should consider actions and rules from a disinterested, dispassionate, omniprecipient, omniscient, consistent point of view.

5. Justice as fairness (Rawls)   The moral agent should consider
                                        rules and actions from the
                                        point of view of the least
                                        fortunate in society.

One can find any of these positions or a combination of them represented in health care settings, whether or not an individual or group examines the explicit assumptions or value positions underlying particular decisions and actions. There are difficulties in appealing to any one position for "the answer" to complex moral problems arising from individual nurse–patient–colleague relationships to policy making for a prepaid group health plan or for population-based health programs.

Vaux, a theologian, has provided us with another model for ethical reasoning and decision making developed from various moral positions. This may be helpful in the *process* of clarifying the issues and value conflicts in a particular situation. This model asks the decision maker to consider and evaluate possible results of decisions-making options on persons involved and to consider side-effects, and possible responses to a given action.[21]

Additional questions to be addressed are: What can be learned from the past that is relevant to this situation, such as, the Nuremberg trials? What do conscience and common sense demand in the present living situation? What makes sense for everyone concerned in this dilemma, for example, a situation requiring a decision about withdrawing treatment? What are the probable consequences of this or that action for the future, for example, telling the truth to a terminally ill patient?[22] Health professionals and others involved may consider all of these questions in seeking to make more rational, thoughtful decisions in the face of complex ethical dilemmas. Echoes of all the ethical positions and theories can be heard in these questions, such as consideration of consequences and respect for the persons involved. Nurses, both as individuals and in collaboration with others, need to consider these questions as they gather information to respond to questions of what is the morally right thing(s) to do in a situation of moral conflict. A key concern is that decisions be made in a more thoughtful, reasoned way, rather than by simply acting on one's gut feeling. Part of learning skills to initiate and participate in these decision-making processes is gaining some familiarity with ethical positions and approaches in the search to determine one' s obligations when there are no ready-made answers.

Nurses might also take a look at recurrent ethical dilemmas in their practice and take action to modify or prevent them from happening. Some recurring dilemmas could be prevented from occurring at the primary level of prevention through listening, careful assessment, and education in dealing with hard choices about treatment in patient, colleague, and family relationships. Such ethical issues as truth-telling, rights of the terminally ill and dying, and experimentation with human subjects better lend themselves to a preventive approach when considered in a noncrisis setting such as in planned ethics rounds, in institutional ethics committees, and in review boards for clinical research proposals.

REFERENCES

1. Callahan D: Normative ethics and public morality in the life sciences. *Humanist* September–October 1972.
2. Frankena WK: *Ethics*, 2nd ed. Englewood Cliffs, NJ: Prentice-Hall; 1973, p 25.
3. Ibid, p 24.
4. Ross D: What makes right acts right? In Sellars W, Hospers J (eds): *Readings in Ethical Theory*. Englewood Cliffs, NJ: Prentice-Hall; 1970, pp 484–485.
5. Frankena WK: *Ethics*, p 29.
6. Ibid, p 30.
7. Kant I: The Metaphysical Elements of Justice. *The Metaphysics of Moral, Part I*. Indianapolis: Bobbs-Merrill; 1965, p 22.
8. MacIntyre A: *A Short History of Ethics*. New York: Macmillan; 1966, p 195.
9. Frankena WK: *Ethics*, pp 39–41.
10. Ibid, pp 42–43.
11. Ibid, p 47.
12. Ibid, p 49.
13. Firth R: Ethical absolutism and the ideal observer. In Sellars W, Hospers J (eds): *Readings in Ethical Theory*. Englewood Cliffs, NJ: Prentice-Hall; 1970, pp 212–214.
14. Ibid, pp 214–218.
15. Ibid, pp 218–221.
16. Rawls J: *A Theory of Justice*. Cambridge, MA: Harvard University Press; 1971, pp 17–22, 62, 136–147.
17. Ibid, pp 136–142.
18. Ibid, p 302.
19. Ibid, pp 131–135.
20. Vaux K: *Biomedical Ethics: Morality for the New Medicine*. New York: Harper & Row; 1974, p 42.
21. Ibid, pp 38–39.
22. Ibid, pp 38–43.

CHAPTER 4

Perspectives on Ethical/Moral Principles

Nurses make judgments that involve human lives and have an impact on the welfare of patients, families, and others. Many of the situations in which such judgments are made involve relationships in which there is conflict between individual needs and values or in which the interests of an individual are in conflict with those of a group. Nurses encounter many situations in their daily work in which ethical questions and concerns require a different order of judgment from what would commonly be considered a clinical judgment, such as when to assist a patient who is ambulating after surgery so as to maximize patient safety and promote appropriate independence. Judgments in the ethical and moral realm are primarily concerned with what is "right" or "good" for patients or for developing policy in areas that raise ethical concern, such as orders not to resuscitate, withdrawal of treatment, or obtaining adequately informed consent. Nurses need more than expert clinical knowledge, which does not automatically transfer into expertise in dealing with the ethical and moral realm. In the process of moral reasoning, nurses may appeal to certain moral rules or principles, such as respect for persons or doing no harm, as justification for taking or not taking certain actions.

Distinctions may be drawn between rules and principles, even though there is no overall consensus as to their exact difference. Principles are considered to be more general than moral rules. Rules are grounded in principles, which serve as foundations for rules.[1] Nurses may appeal to a moral rule, such as the rule that one should never tell a lie. The rule that one should never lie could be grounded in the principles of respect for persons and fidelity or primary loyalty to patients.

Principles may be viewed as governing laws of conduct, as codes of conduct by which one directs one's life or actions, or as generalizations that provide a basis for reasoning. In other words, they provide guidance for decisions and action. They may be grounded in a religious tradition, in secular world views, or in normative ethical theories, such as utility or duties and obligations (discussed in Chapter 3). A principle that is grounded in the formalist or deontological ethical tradition is oriented toward duties and obligations. An example is the nurse's obligation to respect the patients for whom she cares. Part of that obligation is not to tell lies. From a utilitarian viewpoint, respect for persons would be important in making decisions insofar as it has consequences that promote good for the greatest number.

R.M. Hare, a philosopher, reminds us that moral principles are statements that direct or prescribe. He says that a moral principle should suggest or propose certain behaviors that the agent chooses in guiding his or her actions. Moral principles do not directly cause or command particular actions. In this sense, then, a moral principle is an internal suggestion that the nurse uses in guiding behavior rather than a directive made by an external authority figure.[2]

One may or may not be aware of the background theories or grounding of the moral principles one appeals to in making decisions. However, in appealing to them explicitly, one is participating in a principled thinking process that assumes that decisions will have stood the test of consideration in light of principles that meet certain criteria. In a clinical situation that presents an ethical dilemma, principled decisions and actions are assumed, at a minimum, to be reflective of thoughtful and sensitive consideration of what is in the patient's best interests rather than just based on one's own "gut" feelings or unquestioning obedience to the orders of physicians.

Criteria for moral principles have been discussed by philosopher J. Rawls.[3] These are mentioned in Chapter 3 and will be reviewed here for the reader's convenience. First of all, he stated that principles should be general in their application. They should express general properties and relations rather than identify particular persons or associations. In other words, in order to meet the criterion for generality, a principle of respect for persons would not identify physicians and nurses specifically. However, a general principle could be stated so as to hold only for a restricted group, such as pregnant women. Then it would not meet the second criterion of universalizability. That is, principles are to be universal in application. They hold for everyone and are to be chosen in light of the consequences of everyone's compliance with them. Publicity is the third condition to be met. All who are affected by the principle should understand and recognize such a principle. That is, it should be publicly acknowledged and accepted as operational in that society. The fourth condition is that the principle imposes an order on conflicting claims. This condition is not always easy to satisfy but suggests, for example, that appeals to force and threats are unacceptable when making decisions that affect other persons, such as patients. The last criterion is finality. Principles that meet this criterion serve as the final court of appeal. Reasoning from such principles is conclusive, and they are considered even to override what law and custom require. Hence, principled thinking about the ethical dimensions of a decision may lead to the conclusion that the decision is moral and ethical *and* also more than the law or custom demand. Or, the decision may not necessarily be congruent with law at a given place and point in time or conform to custom. An example might be a nurse who argues that he or she has a moral right and even an obligation to tell the truth to a terminally ill patient about her illness under particular conditions in a state where the law is ambiguous and in an institution where the norm is that patients are told by nurses to ask the physician such questions.

ETHICAL PRINCIPLES IN NURSING AND HEALTH CARE

What are some principles that nurses and other health professionals, individually and collectively, use in responding to ethical issues and dilemmas in practice at the patient care level and at the policy-making level? Selected principles discussed here presume the competent practice of each individual delivering nursing care. Ideally, competence is grounded in compassion as the motivating force of the nursing profession.[4]

Consideration of ethical principles in situations that require hard choices suggests the need for a more reflective morality in nursing practice, generally, and in dealing with moral problems that confront nurses and others daily. These situations range from decisions made by and for dying patients in institutional and home settings, to decisions concerning patients in psychiatric settings who refuse treatment, to decisions made about distribution of limited nursing resources in a community where there are elderly, home-bound patients and infants recently discharged from neonatal intensive care units who need nursing care and supervision. These situations raise questions and concerns requiring consideration of such principles as respect for persons, beneficence, and justice in making decisions. The following discussion of these principles is meant to be suggestive rather than exhaustive.

Principle of Respect for Persons

A principle of respect for individuals as persons may be considered to be broader than a principle that speaks simply to assuring the autonomy and self-determination of the individual. In addition to respect for the individual's autonomy, it also recognizes that individuals are members of a human community, which involves consideration (at the same time) that most of the decisions we make affect others. It acknowledges the interconnectedness and interdependence of individuals. This view rejects an extreme ethic of individualism, such as might be used to justify a mildly depressed woman's right to commit suicide simply because she had a right to do as she pleases with her body under an extreme notion of individual self-determination. Respecting the person as an individual *and* as a community member requires consideration of duties and obligations to others as well as to one's self in making decisions.

Respect for the individual requires that each individual be treated as unique and as an equal to every other individual, and that special justification is required for interference with an individual's own purposes, privacy, or behavior.[5] This principle requires that a minimum consideration in decision making affecting an individual is that the individual's own values and goals be considered in any major decisions that affect his present or future welfare. This rules out the paternalistic stance in decision making whereby health professionals or others make decisions for a patient that they consider to be in the patient's best interests, with no consideration of the individual patient's own values and goals. Nurses, individually and collectively, are in a unique interface position between physicians, patients, and families for ensuring that this principle is taken into account in the decision-making process. In some institutions, nurses have already been instrumental in the development of guidelines and policies for "do not resuscitate" orders or care of the dying, which are reflective of this principle.

Commitment to the principle of respect for the individual person would affect whether and how ethical situations were dealt with on a nursing care unit. It would also influence individual nurse–patient and colleague interactions at all levels. Individual nurse–patient interactions and nursing policies would be examined in light of whether they enhanced or negated the principle of respect for both the individual patient and the involved health professional(s). If a patient refused a specific treatment, the nurse would not use coercion to force the patient to accept the treatment but would explore the patient's own goals and values in relation to treatment when the patient is capable of doing so. The nurse would also notify the physician(s) and others involved of the situation and how she or he was dealing with it.

In addition to considering the patient as an individual, the nurse would think about the patient as a person who is a member of a family and community. He or she might appeal to the consequences for others of choices that the patient is considering (such as consequences to a spouse). Nursing action or nonaction is thus justified on the moral basis of whether or not it enhances the uniqueness of the individual, taking into consideration the consequences of choices for significant others, rather than using a legalistic, bureaucratic justification based on "following the doctor's orders" or solely because the patient demands it. Callahan, a philosopher, supports the notion of considering individuals as having obligations as members of families and communities by pointing out the limitations of an extreme individualistic ethic, which he calls "minimalist ethics."[6] Patient or client obligations have not received much attention in current efforts to enhance individual patient autonomy in generally authoritarian health care settings.

Accepting a principle of respect for a person as an individual and as a community member as a general guide to decisions and actions has consequences for the individual patient, for health professionals involved in patient care, and for institutions. Decision making becomes a more time-consuming process in many instances, and there will still be situations where it will be most appropriate for the health professional to make decisions on the basis of the best interests of the patient, such as in a lifesaving type of emergency where the individual is not terminally ill. However, this principle places the burden for justifying why patients should *not* participate in major decisions that affect them on health professionals who automatically make such decisions in the paternalistic, authoritarian structure that exists in many health care institutions. This principle also has implications for how one obtains consent of patients to participate in research and consideration of any possible negative consequences for patients who choose not to participate. Nurses could also consider this and other principles in evaluating organizational structures and relationships among health professionals that impede care that is respectful of persons as individuals in community with others—both patients and caregivers.

Principle of Beneficence

Beneficence may be viewed on a continuum extending from noninfliction of harm or nonmaleficence to benefitting others or positive beneficence. According to Frankena, the principle of beneficence says four things:

1. One ought not to inflict evil or harm.
2. One ought to prevent evil or harm.
3. One ought to remove evil.
4. One ought to do or promote good.[7]

The duty not to inflict evil or harm, or nonmaleficence, takes precedence over the three following aspects, with other things being equal in a situation. However, Frankena says that all are prima facie duties. That is, they are always obligations that one must try to fulfill. They are always to be taken into account, even though there are other considerations that may sometimes outweigh them or take precedence when there is conflict about what action(s) to take. One thinks about such procedures as immunizations for infants. These inflict some degree of pain or discomfort but have long-term health benefits. Or one might consider a surgical procedure, which can be viewed as inflicting harm in order to promote a positive outcome, such as saving a life, diminishing pain and suffering, or increasing mobility. Frankena pointed out that adding the phrase "to or for anyone" to each of the four aspects of beneficence makes this a universalistic principle.

Beauchamp and Childress treat nonmaleficence and beneficence as two separate principles that indicate duties and moral obligations. They do this in part because of the more general understanding of benefi- cence as requiring positive steps.[8] Positive beneficence, as the benefit- ting of others, is frequently invoked as a moral obligation in research where protocols involving sick children are generally of benefit only to future generations. This is one example that illustrates the question as to whether beneficence is a strict moral requirement or an act of charity that is not a moral obligation.

Beauchamp and Childress see nonmaleficence as the prohibition of intentional harm except in special circumstances and as requiring justifi- cation of risks by the probable benefits to be gained. This view is similar to Frankena's discussion. They also take the position that nonmalefi- cence requires that moral agents such as nurses be reflective about their decisions and actions. That is, health care professionals must follow the legal and moral standards of due care, which include knowledge, skills, and diligence.[9]

The beneficence principle requires the provision of benefits and a balancing of harms and benefits.[10] Benefits are considered to have posi- tive value that promotes health or welfare, such as the prevention of illness. Costs, while they are usually thought of in financial terms, can be anything that detracts from human health and welfare, such as phys- ical or psychological pain. Since costs are frequently not quantifiable, they are often referred to as risks. Risks refer to possible future harms. Consideration of risks and benefits by health professionals (and patients or clients) in decision making in treatment and research situations can be considered to be part of the thoughtful and careful action dimension of nonmaleficence. This dimension of beneficence also requires assess- ment and balancing of trade-offs in situations where decisions are often made against a background of uncertainty. A simplistic example is a decision made by a nurse to let a patient sleep an extra hour before awakening him to give a medication when the patient requires both for a positive outcome.

In considering the principle of beneficence before making a deci- sion, one could take the position that nurses are morally required to consider both the possible harm(s) and benefit(s) that might result from a choice to do nothing in a situation of conflict—for example, a physi- cian refusing to discuss a patient's terminal illness with the patient, who then asks the nurse for information. The nurse could choose to ignore the request. Or, the nurse could argue, on this principle, that he or she has a moral right and even an obligation to discuss this with this patient if the nurse knows the "facts," has the necessary communication skills, and has discussed the situation with others involved with the patient. A further moral argument for such action could be based on the principle of respect for the patient as a person and as a fellow member of the human community. To ignore the patient's request would likely produce varying degrees of harm as a consequence.

In situations of conflict, while the principle of beneficence does tell us to promote good while preventing or minimizing harm, it does not give us guidance as to how we are to distribute goods and evils or burdens and benefits when not all will benefit from the required decisions. Such decisions range from determining the number and kind of nursing home beds in a given geographic area to deciding who should get what levels of nursing care in a given institution or in home care when resources are limited. Such decisions require consideration of a principle of justice that might also be reflected in individual nurse–patient relationships where a nurse must decide on allocation of his or her time in an intensive care unit or a community nursing agency.

Principle of Justice

Ideas about justice are basic to the structure of a society and to structures for delivery of nursing and health care. We do not at present have a consensus in our society as to what exactly constitutes justice, although it is recognized that most people have a sense of justice. For example, many health care professionals express concerns about their obligation to deliver quality care when cost containment is a major goal. Distributive justice has to do with the distribution of goods and evils, of burdens and benefits in any society in which resources are limited. It is a matter of comparative treatment of individuals. One needs to consider the morally *relevant* differences between individuals that *justify* differential treatment. There are several suggestions as to what might serve as justification for differential distribution of benefits in such areas as education and health care. These suggestions include contracts, individual need, individual effort, ability to pay, societal contribution, merit, and the idea of equal shares. In actuality, different bases for distribution are used in different contexts. For example, welfare payments are distributed on the basis of need, while jobs and promotions are usually distributed on the basis of achievement and merit.[11]

Individual need is commonly invoked in nursing documents and literature to justify the distribution of nursing and health care. An example is the American Nurses' Association (ANA) Code for Nurses (1985). One issue involved in using need as a basis for just distribution of nursing and health care is who defines needs vis-à-vis demands, wants, and the notion of a fundamental need. A fundamental need for something indicates that a person will be harmed if that thing is not obtained—for example, the need for emergency care if a person is bleeding profusely. It could be argued that decisions for nursing care based primarily on need could be more easily justified in emergency and acute care settings.

Rawls' work on justice as fairness (see Chapter 3) provides one way of looking at a more just distribution of social goods, such as work, income, and self-respect.[12] Fairness is based on consideration of the least advantaged in society in terms of protection of their liberty and opportunity so as to maximize an individual's ability to carry out reasonable life plans. Following Rawls' line of thinking, Daniels has argued that the idea of maintaining normal species functioning provides a possible way to think about a more just way of providing health care and developing policies to do this. According to Daniels, health care needs "are things we need to prevent, maintain, restore, or compensate for departure (such as disease) from normal species functioning."[13] From this, one can argue that there should at least be equal initial access to health care for assessment of the individual's health care needs. While this view has limitations, it is one way of beginning to look more critically at the distribution of scarce nursing resources, which is one aspect of meeting health care needs in our society amid changes such as, technological developments and rationing of health care for the poor and uninsured. This view, then, argues that using income inequalities and ability to pay as screening devices for access to health care is ethically unjustifiable.

These brief discussions of ethical principles and ethical theories (see Chapter 3) are not meant to provide the reader with "formulas" for resolution of ethical dilemmas in practice. In complex nursing care situations where ethical concerns predominate, principles and theories may well conflict. It is hoped that these discussions suggest moral dimensions to be considered in thinking through such situations, in which decisions are made that profoundly affect individuals, families, institutions, and communities. Such considerations will rule out certain options and tell us what is important from an ethical perspective. Toulmin warns us against the tyranny of absolute principles in dealing with real-life situations and problems, as their application can transform painful and intimate moral quandaries into adversarial confrontations.[14] Rather, we are seeking to balance conflicting considerations in the most humane and compassionate way in situations where there are no ready-made answers. Nurses should consider these and other principles, individually or collectively with others, in forums such as ethics rounds and ethics committees when they are confronted with ethical dilemmas in patient or client care and in policy development and evaluation. Such activities are an expression of the principle of fidelity, that is faithfulness and commitment to patients, as a fundamental aspect of the nurse–patient relationship and membership in the community-at-large.[15]

REFERENCES

1. Beauchamp TL, Childress JF: *Principles of Biomedical Ethics*, 3rd ed. New York: Oxford University Press; 1989, p 7.
2. Murphy C: The moral situation in nursing. In Bandman EL, Bandman B (eds): *Bioethics and Human Rights*. Boston: Little, Brown; 1978, p 313.
3. Rawls J: *A Theory of Justice*. Cambridge, MA: Harvard University Press; 1971, pp 130–135.
4. Churchill L: Ethical issues of a profession in transition. *Am J Nurs* 77:874, May 1977.
5. Jonsen A, Butler L: Public ethics and policy making. *Hastings Cent Rep* 5:26, August 1975.
6. Callahan D: Minimalist ethics. *Hastings Cent Rep* 11:19–25, October 1981.
7. Frankena WK: *Ethics*, 2nd ed. Englewood Cliffs, NJ: Prentice-Hall; 1973, p 47.
8. Beauchamp, Childress: *Principles*, p 194.
9. Ibid, p 126.
10. Ibid, p 195.
11. Ibid, p 261.
12. Rawls: *A Theory*, pp 130–135.
13. Daniels N: Cost-effectiveness and patient welfare. In Basson M (ed): *Rights and Responsibilities in Modern Medicine: Ethics, Humanism, and Medicine* (vol. 2) New York; Liss; 1981, pp 162–163.
14. Toulmin S: The tyranny of principles. *Hastings Cent Rep* 11:31–39, December 1981.
15. Aroskar MA: Fidelity and veracity: Questions of promise keeping, truth telling, and loyalty. In Fowler MDM, Levine-Ariff J: *Ethics at the Bedside*. Philadelphia: Lippincott; 1987.

5

Professional Ethics and Institutional Constraints in Nursing Practice

This chapter focuses on the nature of professional ethics in nursing and some of the institutional and social constraints that can act to inhibit the ethical practice of nursing. The discussion will be generally limited to those nurses who practice in hospitals, for two reasons. First, we have more data on this group, and second, over 50% of all employed nurses work in hospitals.

The overriding ethical issue for nurses, especially those working in hospitals, can best be described as one of multiple obligations coupled with the question of authority. As professionals, nurses have a code that maintains that their primary ethical obligation is to the patient. This, in general, means that when an ethical dilemma arises, the nurse places the patient at the center of the dilemma and seeks to discover that patient's ethical stance or what he believes to be in his best interest. The main question is: What does the patient think is the right thing for him in this situation? In some ethical dilemmas, nurses simply want to replace the physician's ethical stance with their own, without either individual having full knowledge of the patient's ethical stance.

Nurses have an ethical obligation to the patient, but they also have an ethical obligation to the physician and to the institution in which they work. As professionals, nurses owe their primary ethical obligation to the patient; however, as employees, nurses also have ethical obligations to the institution and to the physician. To the extent that these multiple ethical obligations mesh so that no conflict develops among them, the nurse should have a clear idea of the right action. However, when conflicts arise between or among these obligations, the nurse has an ethical dilemma. One can argue that nurses are not professionals by certain criteria, but the important fact to remember is that many nurses define themselves as professionals with ethical obligations.

Several examples will help in understanding the concept of multiple obligations better. If the physician makes the decision to withhold information about a patient's diagnosis and prognosis on the basis of his or her best clinical judgment, but the nurses, in their best clinical judgment, believe that the patient should be given this information so that he may function as an autonomous person, the ethical dilemma involving multiple obligations has occurred. Should the nurses go along with the physician and support the decision to withhold information or should they attempt to change the situation so that the patient will know his health status and be able to plan his life accordingly? It will make a difference if there is evidence that the patient does or does not want to know this information.

Further, what should the nurse do in a situation where information has been withheld or distorted by the hospital authorities to prevent a legal suit by the patient's family when a mistake was made in surgery? If the family knows this, they may sue, and such a legal suit, if won, can hurt the hospital's reputation and financial stability. Should the operating room nurse go along with the hospital's definition of events that transpired in the operating room because of her obligation to her employer or should she attempt to have the patient's family told what really happened?

Ethical decisions are usually made in a social context, and that context often has within it constraints that make taking an ethical stance and acting on it a complex matter. The physician has a special legal and ethical relationship with the patient, as well, but as an employee, the nurse also has obligations to the institution and the physician. This social reality of ethics makes being ethical both more difficult in many situations and more complicated. The simple answer to this problem is that the nurse should do what is right and abide by the Code for Nurses. However, an examination of any situation of multiple ethical obligations brings into sharp focus the fact that answers to ethical dilemmas are not usually so easily dealt with.

In the first example given above, the nurse must make a choice between the physician's decision to withhold information and the patient's right to have this information. Let us assume that the physician's stance is based on the ethical principles of nonmaleficence (do no harm) and beneficence (do good) and that he believes that to tell the patient would do harm, since the patient is not emotionally able to cope with the facts of his case. Suppose that the patient has indicated to the nurse that he has some questions about his illness and wonders if he has been told the facts. The nurse, then, becomes concerned about the ethical principle of autonomy and wonders if withholding information from this patient is really not doing harm. She then takes the stance that the patient should be told. Both the nurse and the physician are acting to meet what they think is their ethical obligation to the patient. Yet, it is the nurse who confronts a situation of multiple ethical obligations, obligations to both the patient and to the physician. This is complicated by the fact that the physician is viewed as having more authority to make this type of decision because of his role and his clinical judgment.

When nurses confront situations involving multiple ethical obligations, the first question is: What is the right thing to do, and based on what ethical reasoning? Along with this question, another one comes into play, which is: How far does the nurse's ethical obligation extend? If, in this situation the nurse reasons that the right thing to do is to withhold information, there is no problem of multiple ethical obligations. However, if the nurse does not agree with this decision to withhold information, the second question arises: How far and in what directions does the nurse pursue this obligation to the patient? Should the nurse tell the patient his diagnosis and prognosis? One can argue that this is the ethical and legal obligation of the physician. What if the nurse goes to the physician and explains that the patient is asking for information about his diagnosis and that she thinks that the physician should talk with the patient about this? What if the physician continues with his decision to withhold the information even after the nurse has given him these additional data? Has the nurse met her ethical obligation to the patient? Should the nurse go to other sources, and, if so, which ones? Suppose the nurse goes to the head nurse, but the head nurse does nothing about the situation. Has the nurse's ethical obligation been met? All of these and similar questions stem from two basic questions: (1) what is the nurse's ethical obligation in those situations where she confronts multiple ethical obligations; and (2) what is the extent of this obligation?

NURSING HISTORY AND ETHICS

As far as we can glean from history, the establishment of the first hospital occurred in India before the birth of Christ. Not until the Middle Ages did such institutions develop in Europe. As long as the sick remained at home, their care naturally fell to their families. With the shift from the home to the hospital, the services of some attendants to care for the sick—in addition to the physicians—became a necessity. Early on in this development, two problems regarding these attendants received consideration: (1) how to secure nurses who would provide devoted service; and (2) how to train them to give this service in an efficient manner. The first concern reflects a matter of ethical or religious ideals, while the latter reflects a scientific objective. These considerations, in turn, involve many questions concerning the relationship of nurses to patients and the relationship of nurses to physicians. Both considerations for ethical ideals and scientific objectives, along with the attendant questions regarding the nursing role and how it interacts with the other roles such as the roles of the patient and the physician, remain with us today.

In the early development of these hospital attendants, who would evolve into the nursing professionals we know today, it is unclear whether they were thought of as glorified servants or viewed as professional personnel. In all probability, a mixture of both attitudes coexisted and created a confusion regarding role and function that persisted through many later periods. Women, who constitute over 95 percent of nurses today in the United States, did not enter nursing at this earlier period. The fact that the first nurses were men has been explained by the generally inferior status of women at that time in those places where hospitals developed. The status of women continues to affect nursing in some crucial ways.

Our knowledge of nursing generally goes back to the growth and spread of Christian influence in Europe. At that time, the Church held nursing in high regard and made this known by bestowing sainthood on the nursing leaders. Later, in the sixteenth century, secular trends in nursing began to evolve. The paucity of scientific medicine made the situation such that nurses required no training beyond what could be gained by experience as they worked in the hospital. Nursing practice was, more often than not, a matter of difficult and unpleasant routines. In the past, religious devotion had ennobled this toil and made it worthwhile, but now the religious basis for nursing practice was lacking. For more than three centuries after the Reformation, secular nursing carried with it no promise of a respectable career, and the so-called better types of women tended to avoid it. For many years, nursing was best described as a poorly paid, confining discipline of unpleasant routines, and the typical nurse was depicted as Sairey Gamp, the unpleasant, uneducated, uncouth character in Dickens' *Martin Chuzzlewit*, published in 1844.

The history of nursing in England and the United States since the mid-19th century has evolved from the reforms that Florence Nightingale instituted in nursing education and practice. She maintained that a nursing school should teach the mind as well as form the character. The latter imperative resulted in indoctrination and practice in the middle-class values of the period. Many remnants of the Victorian era and some strands from earlier times remain with us today and reflect the checkered history of nursing, which has included the images of both the saint and the immoral prostitute. One important historical study examining early American nursing points to another factor that has greatly affected the profession. This factor, the systematic oppression of the nursing profession, has affected the quality and delivery of health care.[1]

NURSING ETHICS—A BRIEF BACKGROUND

Many books on nursing ethics in the past have in large part restricted their content to professional etiquette. In 1900, Robb wrote of a breach of etiquette, but her comments reflect the sociology of the situation, including differences in role, function, and status. She remarked that occasionally we find a nurse who, through ignorance or from an increase of her self-conceit and an exaggerated idea of her importance, may overstep the boundary in her relationship with the doctor and commit some breach of etiquette. The point being driven home here is that not only will the individual nurse be made to suffer most acutely, but also her school and the profession at large come in for a share of criticism and blame.[2] More recently, numerous books on ethics have been published for health care professionals in general or specifically for nurses. These books tend to focus on ethical principles and theories.

Aikens, in 1937, devoted two chapters to what she called old-fashioned virtues and included in this category such items as truth in nursing reports, discreetness of speech, obedience, being teachable, respect for authority, discipline and loyalty.[3]

Perhaps one of the most interesting books on nursing ethics, published as a fourth edition in 1943, has a chapter entitled "Master and Servant: Physicians and Nurse." The author says that if the hospital employs the nurse, she is a servant of the hospital and as such the hospital becomes responsible for her acts. With this status, any disobedience to the physician's orders is not only a matter of professional etiquette but a violation of the employee contract. In those situations in which the nurse knows that the physician is mishandling the patient's treatment, she must either continue to carry out his orders or give up the case. This latter choice seems to reflect the fact that many nurses at the time this book was written worked as private duty nurses. The author continues by pointing out that the nurse has no duty to enlighten the public on the relative merits of physicians and the value of their treatment. In short, the nurse ought to remember that she has "a duty of charity as a faithful servant to a master to protect the good name and reputation of the physician under whom she works."[4]

Some years later, another author quoted a remark made by a physician to a nursing school graduating class; he said that to be a successful nurse, one must also be a successful liar. This quote led the book's author into a discussion of loyalty as the nurse's first duty. By virtue of her profession as well as of her implied contract, the nurse owes the physician not only efficient care of patients but also such evidence of loyalty as will strengthen the patient's confidence in him.[5]

All of the above references on nursing ethics were written in this century, and some practicing nurses today read these books or ones similar to them when they were students. Among other things, such input reflects the nature of the socialization process into nursing, the role of women and nurses, and the hierarchical organization in the health care system. Many of these early ethics books delved into the private life and morality of nurses, reflecting the status of nursing students in an apprenticeship system and the stereotype of the intellectually and morally weak woman. Such concerns focused on the individual's morality, and the nurse's duties, obligations, and loyalties referred to a situation in which nurses were, on the one hand, expected to exhibit a dedication of almost a religious nature while, on the other hand, their morality was open to suspicion.[6]

THE NURSING CODE OF ETHICS

The flavor of recent publications reflects some changes in the situation but also contains some threads of continuity from these earlier concerns. The American Nurses' Association (ANA) Code for Nurses outlined in Chapter 1 makes it clear that the nurse's primary commitment is to the patient's care and safety. To fulfill this commitment, the ANA maintains that the nurse must be alert to any instance of incompetent, unethical, or illegal practices by any member of the health team and must be willing to take appropriate actions, if necessary. As to fulfilling this commitment in her own nursing practice, the nurse has the personal responsibility of maintaining competence in practice throughout a professional career. In addition, if a nurse does not believe herself to be competent or adequately prepared to carry out a specific function, she has the right and responsibility to refuse in order to protect both herself and the client.

Any such professional code must, by its very nature, address the general and the ideal, but in doing that it brings to the attention of practitioners the areas of ethical responsibilities, possible areas of ethical conflict, and potential mechanisms for coping with such conflict. In dealing with the general and the ideal rather than the specific and the concrete, a code can only allude to the formal and informal social systems in which practitioners function.

Taking into account historical factors and present realities, four central questions underlie the discussion in the remainder of this chapter. First, can nurses, employed in the bureaucratic system of the hospital, be ethical as outlined in the ANA Code for Nurses? Second, if they practice according to these ethical principles, do they run any risks, and, if so, what are they? Third, do nurses have the right as well as the obligation to provide adequate, if not excellent, nursing care and are they willing and able to exercise this right? Finally, what can the nurse expect from nursing in the way of support if she takes an ethical stance that disrupts some aspect of the hospital norms? These questions will serve to weave together the ideas in the next section on possible constraints that can function at times to inhibit ethical behavior on the part of nurses.

ORGANIZATIONAL AND SOCIAL CONSTRAINTS

One of the most interesting dimensions of hospital nursing arises in the potential for conflicting moral claims on the nurse. Nurses find themselves in situations involving multiple obligations. Until around the time of the Second World War, many, if not most, nurses in hospitals worked as private duty nurses and received a fee for service from the patient. A number of economic and sociological factors converged in the 1930s and 1940s, and this shift away from fee-for-service to hospital-employee status occurred. Whereas previously the nurse's obligation had been to the one patient and the patient's physician, with this shift came a change in occupational status, and the ethics of the situation became more complex. As a hospital employee, the nurse must now balance obligations to the institution, to the attending physician and the house staff, and to the patients themselves while attempting to practice nursing using the ethical code of the profession as a guideline.

Research in the past indicated that nurses believed that their first loyalty belonged to the hospital where they worked. By and large, the potential ethical issues emerging from this situation went without discussion. In the last 20 years, numerous members of the health professions and social scientists have described the roles, role expectations, functions, and status positions of those working in hospitals as well as the social network within which these workers function. Much has been said about the interpersonal and communication problems that arise, but a great deal less has been said about ethical dilemmas except indirectly as they spin off from organization, interpersonal, and communication problems.

As far back as 1964, one such study, which examined baccalaureate students' images of nursing, reported that these students, influenced by faculty members, came to gravitate perceptibly toward individualistic-innovative views of nursing and away from bureaucratic orientations.[7] In a collection of essays, a sociologist also writing in the 1960s described the physician as having a number of different positions that simultaneously provide him with multiple statuses and freedoms from organization control; however, he does have a quasicontractual relationship with the hospital. The sheer power stemming from the free movement accorded to the physician within an otherwise formal bureaucracy sharply contrasts with the role of the nurse, which is profoundly affected by her obligation to represent continuity of time and place. Although the patient care unit becomes her turf, the nurse and the doctor both know that in any direct conflict between them they can be subject to unequal privilege within the system. The implicit threat of the doctor's use of the free-flowing communication prerogative traditionally has put the nurse in a position of having to use flattery, tact, or even subterfuge in her role of coordinator between the entrepreneur and the bureaucratic system.[8] In another essay reflecting the 1960s but relevant in numerous places today, Esther Lucille Brown discusses the hospital organization as a deterrent to professional nursing. She notes a number of factors including the downward communication of frequent orders, rules, and prescribed procedures issued by persons in authority; the often inadequate channels for upward communication of plans, suggestions, and complaints originating on the lower hierarchic levels of nursing; and the problems of limited lateral communication and psychological isolation can decrease initiative and motivation and encourage dependency, feelings of inferiority, and dissatisfaction.[9] In the mid-1970s, the experiences of seven new nurses attempting to innovate inpatient care illustrated some of these problems. They found the nursing administration authoritarian and stifling to the extent that they seemed to hamper improvement in patient care rather than encourage it. These young women asked, "When will nursing administrators let nurses practice as legally indicated in their state's Nurse Practice Act?"[10]

Nurses traditionally have helped doctors in scientific tasks and also helped overcome inadequacies in the scientific method of practicing medicine. Essentially, the nurse has done this by helping to prevent knowledge concerning ambiguities, uncertainties, and errors from reaching the patient and his family. The nurse has been expected to react with moral passivity to her knowledge of hospital events. If she had been a full-fledged professional peer of the physician she would, conceivably, have taken a more active moral stand, whereas she has served more as a sponge and a buffer in the system.

Professionals are part of a moral community. They have social links not only to their clients and colleagues in their own profession but also to other groups whose activities their skills must dovetail. Furthermore, the legitimacy of their professional contribution must be acknowledged by these other groups. By comparison to the professions, the semiprofessional organizations are more bureaucratic and subject to numerous rules governing not just the central work tasks, but extraneous details of conduct on the job. Semiprofessionals do not have a strong reference group orientation to colleagues and do not tend to see the generalized colleague group as a source of norms. Therefore they become more willing to accept an administrative superior as such a source. One reason given for this pattern in the semiprofessions has been the prevalence of women, who are seen to be more amenable to administrative control than men, less conscious of organizational status, and more submissive in this context than men. Such constraints do not tend to make for job satisfaction and can compound the already existing ethical dilemmas. A 1977 survey illustrates this point. Out of 10,000 nurses throughout the country who responded to this survey, 3,800 said that they would not want to be a patient in the hospitals where they worked.[11] Not only did these findings raise serious questions about the quality of hospital care, they shocked some leaders of the nation's hospital industry. Specifically, the survey reported that 18 percent of the respondents said that they knew of deaths caused accidentally by nurses, and 42 percent said that they knew of deaths caused by doctors. Of these nurses, 4 percent reported that they themselves had made mistakes that they believed had led to a patient's death. These findings raise a host of questions regarding the ethical issues in these situations. Such questions come to mind as: How were these situations dealt with ethically? Were formal or informal institutional mechanisms available to consider the ethical aspects of these problem situations?

One typical situation reported by a nurse told of a shortage of nursing personnel on the evening shift in the intensive care unit, where the nurse had responsibility for six patients on ventilators in three separate rooms. This nurse spent about fifteen minutes with one patient who was hemorrhaging and then returned to another room where the patient had accidentally disconnected himself from the machine, arrested, and died. This incident raised the question of human resources and staffing in an area where, by definition, critically ill patients require close attention. What obligation does the nurse have to voice her concern regarding the ethical or legal aspects of this situation? Where would she go with such a concern? Does the nursing service leadership have a moral obligation to try to prevent such an occurrence? One central question basic to all the others has to do with the nature and extent of the professional colleagueship that nurses have with one another and with the nursing service hierarchy. If one nurse raises questions that examine the ethical issues involved in a given situation, whom, if anyone, can she rely on for support in her attempt to practice according to the ANA Code for Nurses? What formal channels need she go through in order to have her concerns heard and seriously considered? At the core of these questions lies the larger question of whether hospital nurses have professional, collegial relationships with one another and whether such a social network can function to provide an arena in which ethical dilemmas can be discussed. As part of this larger question, the role of the nursing leadership must be examined. Given the continuing bureaucratic structure of hospitals, what can the nursing service leadership do to implement the ANA Code for Nurses? How does this leadership view the obligations and rights of the staff nurse? Surely the reported shortage of nurses during the 1980s will have an impact on these questions. An important question that has not received sufficient attention asks: to whom does the nurse administrator owe a primary ethical obligation?

Another finding of this survey suggested that the doctor–nurse game, first described in print in 1967 by Stein, continues to be a factor in the daily routine and decision making.[12] One nurse put it this way: "The conflict itself is not so upsetting as the fact that the patient may have to wait hours or a day before the doctor eventually gets around to ordering what the nurse suggested should be done." A lack of effective communication between doctors and nurses can be a significant factor in explaining poor patient care. Nurses have power when it comes to making decisions about their patients, but they never seem to be giving advice to the doctor. Nurses sometimes pretend they never made diagnoses, although their diagnoses are crucial to the patients' lives.

In another study from the 1970s, nurses perceive physicians as more deficient in communication and participation-encouraging behavior than in directive behaviors. The desired change in physician leadership patterns appears to require change not only in interprofessional behavior but also throughout the system of hospital organization.[13]

As a matter of fact, doctors have not always enjoyed a good reputation in their relationships with coworkers. They tend to regard others as working for them and not for the patient. Despite this delegation of tasks, doctors continue to feel a final medical responsibility, including ethical and legal aspects, for all that happens to their patients. Considerable evidence has been gathered to indicate that the doctor–nurse relationship can be characterized by a fair amount of medical authoritarianism, on the one hand, and nursing's acceptance of dependence or even deference, on the other.[14] This led one nurse educator in the 1970s to say that the most fundamental problem in nursing is its status as a woman's occupation in a male-dominated culture. Even the administrative positions in hospital nursing generally are available only with approval of the male-dominated systems in medicine and hospital administration. She went on to say that nurses who strive never to make a mistake fail to realize that decisions that were never made can be just as wrong as those that were made incorrectly.[15] Wilma Scott Heide, a nurse and an early president of the National Organization for Women, agreed that the problems of nursing are symptoms of the oppression of women.[16] Bullough commented on this situation by pointing out that historically the subordination of women and the sex segregation of nursing and medicine helped to establish interactional patterns between the two professions that included subordination of nurses as well as informal doctor–nurse games. Reinforced by hospital training schools and the state laws that restricted the roles of nurses, these patterns led to stereotyped communication and interaction between nurses and physicians, and this in turn has been a barrier to the full use of the knowledge and skills of nurses. In nursing, those with ambitions for advancement have historically left the bedside, since only by removing themselves from direct clinical involvement can they gain any feeling of autonomy. Certain practice patterns, such as primary care nursing, seem to be changing this. In addition, there are magnet hospitals that draw and keep nurses because they experience job satisfaction. The study on these hospitals identified elements that drew and kept nurses. These elements were in the areas of management, professional practice, and education.[17]

Brown viewed the situation in a similar but broader manner when she pointed out that the health services industry is unusual in that most of the skilled and unskilled workers are women, although the industry is largely controlled by men. Health service occupations are organized like craft unions, with rigid hierarchic separation and control by the top occupation. Conflicts occurring between men and women, between management and workers, often get played out as conflicts between occupations. Because this occupational and sexual segregation overlap, conflict usually revolves around the shape and structure of the occupation and can best be characterized as maneuvering for turf, or, put another way, for control of occupational territory.[18]

A number of factors come together to maintain the situation referred to above. In the past, nursing has drawn into its ranks young women who have had a traditional view of the female role. The picture that emerged was that of conventionally oriented young women who were much more heavily invested in traditional feminine life goals than in career pursuits and reluctant to make more than incidental concessions toward professional involvement. Traditional female socialization remains a major factor in women's work world. It also helps to remind us that the work world has been, for the most part, geared to men and not to women, who often have different home responsibilities. It reminds us too that not only do we lack good child care facilities, but men have been socialized to hold certain ideas about themselves and their wives regarding their respective roles both in the home and outside of it.

At a 1975 research conference, Hall reported on findings from a study in which she compared female nursing students with female medical students. Again, the study found the nursing students expressed a more traditional view of the female role and lacked a career commitment.[19] In short, up to that time, nursing has mostly attracted women with a traditional view of their role, and this has had serious consequences for nursing and has served to maintain the status quo in the decision-making arrangements within hospitals. Some earlier studies also make this point regarding maintenance of the status quo. Whether this continues to be the picture at the present time or not is difficult to say. Certainly more nurses have obtained more education in the last two decades. In addition, fewer nurses work in hospitals than previously reported. Many more clinical settings have become available. All of these factors may mean that more nurses have more career commitments.

In an early study conducted in 1966, researchers designed and executed an experiment in nurse–physician relationships. They believed that the professional status and standards of nurses were challenged at times by the behavior of doctors. They selected the situation in which the doctor directs the nurse to carry out a procedure that, in some fashion, goes against her professional standards. Specifically, they constructed an incident around an irregular order from a doctor to a nurse for her to administer a dose of medication. Essentially, the ingredients of the experimental conflict included: (1) the request for the nurse to give an obviously excessive dose of medicine (since this was a "live" situation, they decided to use a placebo for reasons of safety); (2) the medication order was transmitted by telephone, a procedure in violation of hospital policy; (3) the medication was unauthorized—that is, a drug that had not been placed on the ward stock list and cleared for use; and (4) the order was given to the nurse by an unfamiliar voice. The researchers conducted this conflict situation on 10 wards of a private hospital and 12 wards of a public hospital. One nurse participated per ward, for a total sample of 22 nurses. Of this total, 21 nurses prepared the medication and were walking to the patient with it when they were stopped. In an interview following the conflict situation, a majority of the nurses referred to the displeasure of doctors on occasions when nursing resistance had been offered to instructions that had been considered improper. It has long been recognized that when friction exists between doctors and nurses, it is the patients who chiefly suffer. However, this study underscores the danger to patients in unresolved difficulties of the nurse–doctor relationship even when little or no friction in the usual sense of the word is present. In a situation such as this experimental one, it would be assumed by some that two professional intelligences, the doctor's and the nurse's, were working to make sure that procedures would be undertaken in ways beneficial to the patient. This study has raised some question about that assumption. The authors of this study concluded that a considerable amount of self-deception goes on in the average staff nurse. In nonstressful moments, when thinking about her performance, the average nurse tends to believe that considerations of her patient's welfare and of her own professional honor will outweigh considerations leading to an automatic obedience to the doctor's orders at times when these two sets of loyalties come into conflict.[20] It would be helpful to repeat this study to see if the findings would be the same today. However, this is deceptive research in that the nurses did not know they were in a study and did not give informed consent, so such a protocol would have difficulty at the review for safeguarding the rights of human subjects. There are other research methodologies that could assist us to explore this question and update our understanding of these important questions about gender, role, and professional socialization.

The official view of the nursing profession has been that the nurse will habitually defend the well-being of her patient as she sees it and strive to maintain the standards of her profession. This study surely counts among its implications the idea that professional relationships between nurse and doctors may exert a limiting effect upon the nurses' resourcefulness and, in some cases, increase the hazard to which the patients undergoing treatment are exposed. The trust and efficiency that the nurses demonstrated in the above study are qualities that, in their place, can be of inestimable value to physicians and patients. Obviously, the nursing and medical professions need to find ways in which these and other traditional values can be reconciled with the nurse's fuller exercise of her intellectual and ethical potentialities.

Before completing this discussion on organizational and social constraints, special notice must be given to the concept of paternalism. In his essay *On Liberty*, Mill wrote that ". . . the sole end for which mankind are warranted, individually or collectively, in interfering with the liberty of action of any of their number, is self-protection. . . . He cannot rightfully be compelled to do or forbear because it will be better for him to do so, because it will make him happier, because, in the opinion of others to do so would be wise, or even right." What Mill is essentially saying is that we cannot advance the interests of the individual by compulsion, or, if we attempt to do so, the evil involved outweighs the good done. Mill believed that the individual person could best serve as judge and appraiser of his own welfare, interests, needs, and so forth. Others, including fellow Utilitarians, have vigorously attacked this claim on the grounds that little proof exists to indicate that most adults are well acquainted with their own interests.[21]

Paternalism can be thought of as the use of coercion to achieve a good that is not recognized as such by those individuals for whom the good is intended. Because coercing a person for his own good denies him a status as an individual entity, Mill strongly objected to paternalism and did so in absolute terms. To be able to choose is a good that is independent of the wisdom of what is chosen, or, as Mill put it, a person's mode of laying out his existence is the best, not because it is the best in itself, but because it is his own mode. Mill's position has some problems in it, which remain beyond the scope of this discussion; however, for him paternalism became justified only to preserve a wider range of freedom for the individual in question.

The concept of paternalism, as used in the medical ethics literature, most often refers to the attitudes and behaviors of the physician toward the patient. However, Ashley, in her historical study mentioned earlier, documented that paternalism on the part of doctors and hospitals has resulted in serious and systematic injustice against women in the health sciences that has been both morally indefensible and socially damaging. She developed her thesis by pointing out that medicine and nursing have not constituted a complementary pair of professional groups sharing common interests and goals. Although they developed in close proximity, this has not resulted in cooperative activity for the good of the patient. In large part, this situation resulted from the paternalism in medicine—paternalism, in this case, laced with prestige and power. A recent example of medical paternalism can be found in the American Medical Association's attempt to create a new category of worker, the Registered Care Technician, to combat the impact from the nursing shortage. This action was undertaken in a unilateral fashion without consultation with the American Nurses' Association. Such a situation placed the nursing association on the defensive and caused it to spend time, money, and energy on trying to defeat the establishment of this new worker in the clinical setting.

A 1980 study conducted by Mabel Wandelt, reported in The *American Nurse*, examined the factors that cause nurses to leave nursing.[22] The major cause was undesirable working conditions. Specifically, these undesirable conditions included a lack of administrative support by hospital and nursing service administrators. When conflicts arise between a nurse and a physician, the administrators frequently ". . . side with the physician. They just don't support nurses." Lack of autonomy, inflexibility of working hours, and being pulled from a familiar unit to be placed temporarily on a short-staffed unit were cited by the 3500 nurses who returned the questionnaire. Other difficulties included child and family schedules, frequent overtime with no additional compensation, personnel, and low salaries. Although salary was a factor in these findings, nurses ranked this seventh among the reasons why inactive nurses were not working. The important factor driving people out of nursing was the tension of not having a say over their own actions and not having confidence that patients were receiving safe care. In 1981 the National Commission on Nursing conducted public hearings and published a report. Four of the five problems most frequently mentioned were: (1) the status and image of nursing; (2) the effective management of nursing resources including staffing, scheduling, and salary; (3) the relationship among nursing staff, medical staff, and hospital administration; and (4) the maturing of nursing as a self-determining profession.[23]

These conditions that lead to job dissatisfaction for nurses raise many questions about the ethics of care, as well as questions about the ethical obligations of nurse administrators as mentioned earlier. At the base line, the central question has to do with the multiple ethical obligations that nursing administrators confront and how they deal with them. What are the administrator's ethical obligations toward the nursing staff and how can these be met in the hospital environment? In addition, is there support not only from the administration but from nursing peers as well? This raises the question as to how nurses can work together professionally to deal effectively with ethical dilemmas that arise in their daily practice.

This chapter has raised questions regarding the second level and has focused on the possible organizational and social constraints in hospitals that may act to impede the ethical practice of nursing. Several interrelated themes have been developed and include the role and social position of the physician and the nurse in the hospital's social system, the bureaucratic nature of that system, the role and power of the nursing leadership in the system, sexism, and paternalism. In addition, the traditional female sex role socialization, which may have been reinforced by some nursing school values, favors passivity in many matters, including those of an ethical nature. In the extreme, it leads to the Nazi mentality, where one does a good job by simply following orders. All of these factors combine to maintain the status quo.

The crucial questions for the nurse concerning ethical dilemmas are: Given these factors, can the nurse be ethical? Is one factor the task of becoming aware of the ethical, as well as the clinical, aspects of nursing situations? Does one need to think through one's own values and ethical stances? What in the system can help the nurse to act on her values and ethical stances? Would a formal mechanism of staff discussion help? Could some structural mechanisms be developed to provide colleagueship within the nursing ranks and between the staff and the leadership levels? Do nurses have a right as well as an obligation to attempt to practice according to the ANA Code for Nurses? Do they want to invest that much? The remainder of this book assumes that nurses do want to be guided by moral considerations in their professional activities, and to that end the following chapters discuss some central ethical dilemmas and nursing practice. But first, a brief discussion of formal mechanisms as an arena in which ethical dilemmas can be discussed is useful.

MECHANISMS FOR DISCUSSING DILEMMAS

Ethics rounds are an excellent medium in which to discuss ethical dilemmas. These rounds are similar to any other nursing or medical rounds, except that the clinical data become background material necessary to focus on the ethical dilemmas. The various formats for and possible participants in ethics rounds have been discussed elsewhere.[24-26] Every health care facility interested in having ethics rounds will need to work out the details to fit its particular situation.

Many hospitals and other health facilities have an ethics committee established to deal with those clinical ethical dilemmas that have not been worked out at the ward level. From observation of such committees, it is apparent that they function most effectively when a variety of people are members. Such categories of health professionals as hospital administrator, lawyer, nurse, physician, hospital chaplain, social worker, and bioethicist, if one is available, together bring a wealth of information and perspectives to the issue at hand. The extent to which an ethics committee will be effective will depend on the chair and members, whether the committee itself and others take the committee seriously, and how the committee meets its charge. Such a committee is one obvious place of interaction between the ethical and the political.[27-37]

In addition to the development of clinical ethics committee, some institutions have also established a nursing ethics group to address the ethical issues of nursing practice. Such a forum examines ethical problems that relate specifically to nursing and explores ethical choices nurses consider and make on a daily basis.[38,39]

If your place of work does not have a clinical ethics committee or has one without nursing representation, you and some of your colleagues may want to change that. Also you may find a nursing ethics group a useful arena in which to discuss the ethical dilemmas you confront.

REFERENCES

1. Ashley JA: *Hospitals, Paternalism, and the Role of the Nurse.* New York: Teachers College Press; 1976.
2. Robb IH: *Nursing Ethics.* Cleveland: Koeckert; 1900, p 250.
3. Aikens CA: *Studies in Ethics for Nurses,* 4th ed. Philadelphia: Saunders; 1937, pp 74–92.
4. Moore DTV: *Principles of Ethics,* 4th ed. Philadelphia: Lippincott; 1943, Chap 13.
5. McAllister JB: *Ethics with Special Application to the Medical and Nursing Professions,* 2nd ed. Philadelphia: Saunders; 1955.
6. Deloughery GL, Gebbie KM: *Political Dynamics: Impact on Nurses and Nursing.* St Louis: Mosby; 1975, Chap 9.
7. Davis F, Olesen VL: Baccalaureate students' images of nursing. *Nurs Res* 13:8–15, Winter 1964.
8. Mauksch HO: The organizational context of nursing practice. In Davis F (ed): *The Nursing Profession.* New York: Wiley; 1966, pp 109–137.
9. Brown EL: Nursing and patient care. In Davis F (ed): *The Nursing Profession,* New York: Wiley; 1966, pp 176–203.
10. Genn N: Where can nurses practice as they're taught? *Am J Nurs* December 74:2212–2215, 1974.

11. Hospital nurses in a poll report needless deaths. *New York Times*, January 9, 1971, p 21.
12. Stein LI: The doctor–nurse game. *Arch Gen Psychiatry* 16:699–703, 1967.
13. Bates B, Chamberlin RW: Physician leadership as perceived by nurses. *Nurs Res* 19:534–539, November-December 1970.
14. Bates B: Doctor and nurse: Changing roles and relations. *N Engl J Med* 288:129–134, July 16, 1970.
15. Cleland V: Sex discrimination: Nursing's most pervasive problem. *Am J Nurs*, 71:1542–1547, August 1971.
16. Heide WS: Nursing and women's liberation: A parallel. *Am J Nurs*, 73:824–827, May 1973.
17. McClure ML, Poulin MA, Sovie MD, Wandelt MA: *Magnet Hospitals*. Kansas City: MO, Am. Academy of Nsg. 1983.
18. Brown CA: Women workers in the health service industry. *Int J Health Serv* 5:173–184, 1975.
19. Hall B: Comparative study of female nursing students and female medical students. Paper presented at the Western Interstate Council of Higher Education in Nursing Research Conference, Phoenix, AR, Spring, 1975.
20. Hofling CK, et al.: An experimental study in nurse–physician relationships. *J Nerv Ment Dis* 143:171–180, 1966.
21. Hart HLA: *Law, Liberty and Morality*. Stanford, CA: Stanford University Press; 1963.
22. Work conditions cause nurses to leave. *Am Nurse* November-December 1980, pp 1, 19.
23. National Commission on Nursing: *Initial Report and Preliminary Recommendations*. Chicago: Hospital Research and Educational Trust; 1981, p 10.
24. Davis AJ: Ethics consultation with hospital employees in complex medical settings. In Fletcher JC, *Ethics Consultation in Health Care*. Ann Arbor, MI: Health Administration Press; 1989, pp 109–116.
25. Davis AJ: Helping your staff address ethical dilemmas. *J Nurs Admin* 12:9–13, February 1982.
26. Glover JJ, Ozar DT, Thomasma DCS: Teaching ethics on rounds: The ethicist as teacher, consultant and decision maker. *Theo Med*, July 1986, pp 13–32.
27. Freedman B: One philosopher's experience on an ethics committee. *Hastings Cent Rep*, 11:20–22, November 1981.
28. Younger S, Jackson DL, Coulton, C: A national survey of hospital ethics committees. *Crit Care Med*, 11:902–905, November 1983.
29. Brennan TA: Ethics committees' discussion to limit care. *JAMA* 253:803–807, August 1988.
30. Lo B: Behind closed doors: Promises and pitfalls of ethics committees. *N Engl J Med*, 305:46–50, July 2, 1987.
31. La Puma J: Ethics by committee? *N Engl J Med*, 305:1418, November 26, 1987.
32. Macklin R: The inner workings of an ethical committee. *Hastings Cent Rep*, 18:15–25, March 1988.
33. Siegler M: Ethics committees: Decision by bureaucracy. *Hastings Cent Rep*, 16:22–24, June 1986.
34. La Puma J, Toulmin SE: Ethics consultants and ethics committees. *Arch Intern Med*, 149:1109–1112, May 1989.

35. Grillot A, Davis AJ: Ethical dilemmas—Establishing an ethics committee. *Nurs Success Today*, 3:4–7, May 1986.
36. Jaeger TB: A head nurse's approach to multidisciplinary ethical conferences. *Nurs Manage*, 19:60, 62, January 1988.
37. Harris S: Ethics committees: An inside look at how they function. *Provider*, 12:34–35, July 1986.
38. Edwards BJ, Haddad AM: Establishing a nursing bioethics committee. *J Nurs Admin* 18:30–33, March 1988.
39. American Hospital Association: The nursing ethics group: When the ethics committee is not enough. *Hosp Ethics*, 5:15–16, January-February 1989.

CHAPTER 6

Rights, Obligations, and Health Care

Rights *and* obligations of both patients and nurses are of concern to nurses as they seek to meet individual needs and to act as patient advocates in health care organizations where cost containment continues to be a major goal. One dimension of cost containment that is not yet widely recognized is that taking patient rights such as self-determination seriously through patient involvement in treatment decision making gives better patient outcomes while using fewer resources.[1] Nurses and nursing services are key players in such efforts.

The focus for the past two decades has been on patient rights, with little attention paid to patient obligations. Increasing emphasis on patient or client responsibilities and obligations in health care has caused this focus to shift to some degree. One example is the emphasis on personal responsibility for one's health and for the moderation of health risks that can be changed through healthier behaviors. More attention is also being paid to the rights, as well as responsibilities, of nurses and how they are linked with the enhancement of quality patient care and a sense of moral adequacy in practice.[2]

The American Nurses' Association (ANA) Code for Nurses with Interpretive Statements (1985) uses "rights" language. These "rights" include safeguarding "the client's right to privacy," a major value in our individualistic society. This right is interpreted as an inalienable right of all persons and is what might be considered a basic human right in health care. Several rights of clients are mentioned in the interpretation of Statement I in the Code, which addresses nurses providing services to clients based on respect for human dignity and the uniqueness of the client. Clients have moral rights to determine what will be done with their own bodies, to be given information that is necessary for making decisions, to be told the possible effects of care (including nursing care), and to accept, refuse, or terminate treatment. The ANA document entitled *Nursing: A Social Policy Statement* (1980) mentions access to opportunities for growth and possible change as every person's rights in addressing nursing's concern for health as a means to meaningful and manageable life. Rights, in these views, are far-reaching and have implications for many nursing actions and for the advocate role claimed by nurses and other providers. They must also be considered in the wider context of "rights" discussions in health care and the increasing emphasis on personal responsibility for one's health.

CONCEPTS OF RIGHTS

Rights and obligations of individual persons emerge within the relationships of a human community and can be thought of in several ways. Our society has changed dramatically during the past two centuries from a society that emphasized the obligations of citizens to one that has focused more recently on the rights of citizens and the protection of these rights. The list of rights claimed in today's world is almost endless. Rights, as entitlements, are claimed *to* privacy, to life, to death, to a healthy environment, and to health care. Special rights *of* various groups, such as children, the poor, and the elderly are also claimed. Jellinek provides one explanation of the more recent emphasis on rights claims in health care. He said that patient trust is eroded in large impersonal medical centers and gave examples of this in patient–institution relationships and arrangements, such as lack of continuity of care and frequent violations of confidentiality.[3]

Rights language may also be used to indicate areas where social change is needed in order to move toward a more just system, as in the civil rights movement. This focus on rights in health care is changing as more emphasis is placed on primary prevention and the individual's responsibility for his or her own health as health status relates to lifestyle choices.

There are many views about what constitutes a right and about different types of rights. Yet, the underlying notion of rights is grounded in respect for persons within a social context. Bertram Bandman, in writing about human rights, said that they are moral rights of fundamental importance. They are more important than any other rights and are shared equally by all human beings, in this instance, patients and nurses. They override all other rights that conflict with them. If one is deprived of human rights, there is a grave affront to justice.[4] Many human rights are negative rather than positive rights, such as the right not to be tortured. The United Nations Declaration of Human Rights supports the existence of basic human rights.

Another view of rights says that individuals derive rights from natural law, which has its source in the Greek tradition of justice—that is, the law of the cosmos as necessary, inevitable, and eternal to be discovered through reasoning. This divinely ordered Platonic universe eventually merged with the Judaic concept of the world and natural rights created by God, the lawgiver. Natural law as a source of rights says that there are natural, universal, and inalienable rights of persons as part of nature.[5] The origin of rights in this tradition is grounded in metaphysics and theology. Some authors claim that the only way to know what these alleged natural rights are is through the use of human reason. Others appeal to divine revelation. Both appeal to the idea that rights are discovered rather than created by human beings.

A modern world view maintains that rights are derived from the state and ordered by law—a more limited and legalistic view of rights. While such documents as the United Nations Declaration of Human Rights claim that there are fundamental human rights, including health-related rights, which all people should enjoy, the assertion of rights does not mean they exist automatically in the legal sense or that they are exercised in a society.

Rights have been viewed as powers, claims, or privileges to which one is entitled. Many concepts of rights such as women's rights or rights to health care are entwined with a given social system and its legal subsystem, since rights may be considered as legitimate claims to something and claims against someone or something, such as a hospital or an individual.

RIGHTS AND OBLIGATIONS IN HEALTH CARE

Legally, a right has to do with the power of an individual to change something or to keep it the same, such as a contractual relationship for health care. Distinguish rights from claims, because they are often confused, Curran, an expert in health law, suggests that a claim is a right governing the actions of another person in relation to one's person or property. An example of such a claim is an individual's right not to be assaulted by a physician while receiving medical treatment.[6] The other side of a claim is a duty or an obligation. In the example given, the physician has the obligation not to assault the patient and a duty to avoid harm; a patient has a right to safe nursing care while in the hospital and the nurses employed by the hospital have a corresponding legal and moral obligation to provide safe care. This notion of rights is distinct from a privilege, which is a benefit or advantage given to you by someone else, as in joining an exclusive club. In claiming a right within the legal system, one must seek an answer to questions of whether or not something is actually endangered, such as one's person or property, and who, if anyone, has an obligation to honor the claim.

The Constitution of the United States sets forth what people may generally expect from the federal government, such as the purposes and functions of government, the relationship with state governments, and some notion of what individuals must give up in order to preserve the interests and safety of everyone. Constitutional amendments speak more distinctly to rights or protection of individuals or groups from governmental interference, providing citizens with a very broad sweep of "rights." Constitutional amendments are appealed to in cases where rights of citizens are challenged, such as cases involving civil rights. There is no Constitutional amendment specific to health or health care. According to Macklin, the philosopher Hart distinguishes between special and general rights.[7] He says that special rights are those that arise out of particular transactions or relations between persons in the transaction. In these transactions, rights and duties exist only between the participants, as in physician–patient relationships or the child–parent relationship. General rights, according to Hart, are those that arise out of a principle of equity, that all persons equally have the right to be free—that is, a person may not be unjustifiably coerced. When a conflict of individual rights occurs, such as in a nursing home where two nursing home roommates claim a right to privacy and demand a private room, one person's freedom is necessarily limited by that of the other since residents do not have unlimited access to a private room on demand. This reality limits the freedom of those who do not have access to health care because they are uninsured and confirms that general rights to health care do not exist. Hart's discussion of special and general rights still does not provide us with justification for making claims about individual rights. One could review, however, policies of a health care organization or treatment of nursing home residents or hospital patients in light of whether they include adequate protection of individual autonomy and safety. In addition to moral and legal rights, there are intermediate rights. These are rights that, if taken into a court of law, would in all likelihood be recognized as legal rights. Some think that equitable access to health care might fall into this category of intermediate rights.

Macklin, a philosopher and bioethicist, maintains that some of the debates and uncertainties about rights would be resolved to some extent if we had a framework provided by an overall theory of justice within which such debates could be decided. One example might be Rawls' theory of justice as fairness, whereby the least advantaged in our society must receive some benefit from social and health policies that are developed. The impact of governmental policies on society's most vulnerable would have to be considered in all policy development, and the burdens of a policy could not fall solely on the least advantaged, such as the elderly poor or children. Lacking a social consensus on an overall theory of justice, it is difficult to justify specific rights in our society, such as a right to health care. However, claims to rights may still serve "as expressions of moral outrage or as demands for social and legislative reform."[8] This use of the term *rights* is illustrated in legislation about patient rights, such as the use of written advance directives for medical treatment if one is unable to make one's own decisions or to share in decision making about medical treatment.

In asserting certain rights in health care, one should recognize that this is only one way of placing issues within an ethical framework. One may also consider the deontological approach, which stresses duties and obligations, or the utilitarian approach, which looks at consequences of actions in terms of utility and the greatest good or the least suffering for the greatest number of people. Often framing an issue solely in terms of rights, with no consideration of responsibilities, further confuses the issue, makes for adversarial confrontations, and does not provide clarification or resolution. This is the case when individual rights, such as a right to health care, are claimed that are difficult to substantiate. Another difficulty is that a person can justifiably claim to possess a right even though that claim is currently unprotected by law or social custom. This is an example of an unrealized right. Unrealized rights are "claims" to something not recognized by society. This is the case with some claims of rights in health care. If there were a realized right to health care, it would imply that health care professionals should provide care to those who want it.[9] This is an expression of a correlative obligation.

Macklin warns that there are many moral and philosophical problems in the attempt to discover where rights come from and in whom they reside, even though they are so often appealed to in public debate and in making demands for action of a particular kind, such as access to health care.[10] In attempting to translate rights into correlative obligations, she says that not all of the health, care obligations derived from the rights claimed by some persons or groups can be delivered.[11] Macklin's point is well taken when one considers the ethical issues that arise when the rights to health care of particular groups and individuals come into conflict at the time the health services are actually delivered. Should the latest medical technologies be provided for a middle class child and little or no primary care be provided to the child whose parents are poor and have no health care insurance coverage? Can an obligation be derived solely from the poor child's needs for care? One could argue in the affirmative if one uses a notion of distributive justice grounded in individual needs for medical care, that is, the criterion of medical necessity. Another example of obligations arising from sources other than rights of individuals or groups is the obligation of nurses to provide competent nursing care. These obligations arise for the individual who has the knowledge base of a profession that provides a socially valuable service. Nurses are in a special relationship with patients. This relationship carries with it explicit obligations for the nurse to act in particular ways, such as performing nursing procedures safely and treating patients with respect for their individual dignity.

For purposes of this chapter, following Macklin's thinking, the concept of rights will be used to indicate some legitimate expectations of persons in a given society at a given time. It may be more useful to think of claims about rights not as things to be discovered as true or false but as language used to promote change and social legislative reform. Rights do not assert anything about the moral order per se, but the idea that jeopardizing human rights is an affront to justice is compelling. Many would agree that human rights include a right to health care as a necessary means to carrying on one's life. If this is the case, the fact that not all people have access to health care is ethically unacceptable.

If one claims a right to health care, to whom does one present the claim? Physicians? Government? Insurers? Is there a corresponding moral obligation on the part of some individuals or institutions to provide persons with health care? Part of the problem in responding to such a claim lies in our definitions of health itself. Health is a slippery term, even when one thinks of it as absence of illness or the ability to carry on daily activities. The World Health Organization's concept that health is a "state of complete physical, mental, and social well-being" does not give much direction when considered in the light of rights claims, development and implementation of public policy, and the limitless economic burdens that an attempt at its realization would entail for society. It provides no boundaries within which to consider obligations to provide health care. Health per se is not always a top social priority, even as the means to other ends. The concept of a right to health care also runs into difficulty when one starts talking about individual responsibility for one's life-style choices, especially when those choices involve known risk factors.

The shift to a focus on obligations in health care is illustrated in the report entitled *Securing Access to Health Care*, issued by the President's Commission for the Study of Ethical Problems in Medicine and Biomedical and Behavioral Research.[12] This report concludes that society has an ethical obligation to ensure equitable access to health care. The focus has clearly shifted from a rights orientation in and to health care. Equitable access, as discussed in the Commission report, refers to everyone having access to some level of health care, that is, "enough care to achieve sufficient welfare, opportunity, information, and evidence of interpersonal concern to facilitate a reasonably full and satisfying life."[12] Inherent in these societal obligations is the notion of the special importance of health care in relieving suffering and in demonstrating mutual empathy and compassion for all citizens. This shift may reflect the renewed concern for our interdependence and interconnectedness in community, which has been largely neglected in the societal emphasis on the value of individualism that is only one side of the many-faceted coin of lived reality. Individuals are not absolutely autonomous and isolated. Even the idea that the exercise of individual rights includes corollary obligations negates a perspective of radical individualism.

Callahan suggests that the "right to health care" as a social obligation might be undertaken by a society in terms of equal access to available health care and facilities.[13] While this seems reasonable on the face of it, such a concept has difficulties because of the competition of health with other welfare rights and with other societal values such as the need for education and defense. Debates rage as to whether children and the elderly have the same rights to health care and whether or not those who choose life-styles that put them at risk should have equal access to health care at public expense. Drug abusers and smokers come to mind. An added complexity in dealing with this issue is that we cannot yet explain *why* individuals have undesirable health habits. Since there is little empirical data to help in the resolution of these issues, there is no empirically established foundation that serves to guide development of health policy. Another possible solution to the dilemmas involved in rights arguments for health care is embodied in the concept of legislating universal health insurance or a national health plan for the United States.

The concept of a right to *medical* care underlies Medicare and Medicaid legislated in the 1960s. A strong opposing view to medical care as a right is presented by Sade, a physician. He claimed that man has a primary right, the right to lead his own life.[14] As a consequence of this right, physicians should not be coerced into government schemes that require their services. If physicians are forced to meet this governmental obligation, they have lost personal liberty and the personal freedom to decide how they will practice medicine. This position seems to assume that physicians have no obligations to society even though society legitimizes their practice as a socially valuable service. It also assumes that only physicians will have freedom curtailed to some degree by making medical care a right as a matter of public interest and policy. Again, this position points up the conflict between rights as claims of individuals and the welfare of all—that is, the claimed right of physicians to treat whom they wish and the unrealized rights of all to some adequate measure of health care. This question is by no means settled, as various efforts are made by government to control health care costs, including controls on reimbursement to physicians, and to devise ways to provide health care to the uninsured and underinsured. There are also underlying arguments about whether health care professionals have *rights* to practice or are granted the *privilege* of practicing.

The argument could be made that if it is the obligation of both the public and private sectors, with the federal government as ultimately responsible, to provide health care, then individuals have obligations not only to obtain care but to consider the influence of their own life-style choices on personal health and the welfare of others. Just putting more money into *medical* care is not the solution to some of the health problems in our society, such as alcoholism and AIDS. Availability of and access to medical care must be balanced with individual responsibility for health maintenance. Illich points to the undesirable dependence of individuals on the medical care system—its care and drugs—the "medicalization of life."[15] A broad view of health suggests that rights to health care and the fostering of health should include attention to such "preconditions" of health as general environmental conditions, for example, clean air, clean water, adequate housing, and income adequacy, all of which contribute to health status.[16] These are the life support systems of all of us. They may be even more important factors in determining health status for many individuals and communities than more medical care facilities or development of reimbursement schemes that pay for more medical care. This is an argument for both societal and personal responsibility for health of adults and children.

The report of the President's Commission on *Securing Access to Health Care* concludes that society has an obligation to provide all citizens with an adequate level of care without excessive burdens.[17] It goes on to state that the costs of achieving equitable access ought to be shared in a fair way. Efforts to contain rising health care costs, while important, should not focus on limiting access for the least well-served people or the most vulnerable. Taking such a concept seriously means that some state efforts to set priorities for Medicaid funding are ethically questionable because of their impact solely on the poor. Cost-containment efforts, such as those mandated by the federal government in policy actions such as Diagnosis Related Groups (DRGs) as the basis for hospital reimbursement, are driving decision making. The evidence to date is that these efforts have not contained costs. Simultaneous with the increased attention to costs of health care is increased concern for quality of care and ensurance of quality through assessing outcomes of patient care. All of these activities have an impact on patient rights and obligations. As our society struggles to meet health care needs, particularly those of the uninsured or underinsured, we are reminded of Macklin's point, that we have difficulty in determining what rights are and how they originate because we have no overall theory of justice to provide a societal framework in which legitimate rights can be claimed.

A further challenge still remains. That challenge is to determine what constitutes an adequate level of health care. This is complicated by claims of "needs" that would have been considered luxuries a generation ago in our society. If one does appeal to needs as a standard for making medical care available, whose definition of needs serves as the criterion? *Needs* and *demands* represent two very different concepts in looking at claims to rights for care. Is the health care system obligated to meet uninsured individuals' demands for use of all available health care technologies? How should health care professionals and consumers decide what needs are to be met in providing an adequate level of health care? Callahan claims that in order to make such determinations, we must, as a society, consider what are the appropriate goals of health and priorities for health care.[18] He suggests that the first priorities should be caring activities such as caring for the chronically ill and broad public health measures that include prevention and decreasing morbidity. Curing the disease of individuals would then not be the first priority in health care.

Generally, under common law, the public has no legal right to medical care from private health care providers. However, the Manlove case in Delaware established that private hospitals do incur legal obligations to the community by offering care and having an emergency room. The hospital meets a public need and offers a public benefit.[19] This has been very difficult to enforce in reality. Even government involvement in the form of Hill-Burton funds and federal tax exemptions to hospitals does not necessarily ensure every individual access to care in a particular hospital. The federal government has been forced to establish legislation that forbids the "dumping" of patients from one hospital emergency room to another because of lack of reimbursement.

One way to have enforceable rights to medical care is through a private contract for reimbursement in the form of health insurance. Unfortunately, even if one has health insurance or belongs to a managed care plan such as a health maintenance organization, all costs associated with medical care are not covered and often one's choice of provider is limited. Health maintenance organizations have achieved varying degrees of success in delivering cost-effective health care. Some have floundered and failed whereas others are meeting their goals to provide cost-effective quality care to their members. Some insurance plans still provide incentives for hospitalization rather than ambulatory care services. With more acutely ill patients being discharged from hospitals now than in the past, there is an enormous need to develop and finance long-term care and home care services, particularly for the uninsured and underinsured.

PATIENT RIGHTS AND OBLIGATIONS IN HEALTH CARE

Historically, the movement for patients' rights came out of the Welfare Rights Organization and demands for rights for the disadvantaged in the late 1960s. The overall goals of what has been called the Patients' Rights Movement had to do with quality of health care, the improvement of care, and having some impact on health care providers in changing the system to make it more answerable to patient needs. More specifically, many individuals are seeking more self-determination and control over their own bodies when hospitalized in a paternalistic system that is often still characterized by professional dominance, complicated bureaucracies, endless red tape, and authoritarianism. In this area, one sees clearly the tension between what professionals consider to be their obligations or rights to provide care in the way they feel would be most beneficial to patients, the patient's right to self-determination, and constraints on payment for patient care. The issues of confidentiality, informed consent and decision making, and patient rights to refuse particular kinds of treatment all reflect the conflict between the respective duties and rights of providers and consumers. This theme is carried through all chapters of this book.

Patients are protected against assault and battery by the law of torts (injury or wrongful acts), but when it comes to such areas as informed consent and truth telling, the issues are not as clear-cut in any particular patient care situation that is complex and dynamic. For example, how does one provide adequate information for informed patient decision making? What does one tell a patient about the risks of a particular medical procedure? The standard used is what the reasonable patient needs to know to make a decision about treatment; it is a *process* of education. Informed consent is not simply a matter of having the patient sign a form. Who defines the reasonable patient? A physician? An ethics committee? A family? A community? The rights of patients to participate in decision making are particularly difficult to determine with mental health clients, young children, and those declared incompetent by some stated criteria. The President's Commission discussed the assessment of decision-making capacity as a responsibility of health care providers, since the determination of legal competence is not an issue in most patient decision-making situations.

A further problem to be considered in claiming patient rights in health care is the imbalance of power in patient–physician, nurse–patient, or patient–provider–payer relationships. This imbalance is obvious in the paternalism underlying some of the items in the American Hospital Association Statement (AHA) on a Patient's Bill of Rights (1972). The patient traditionally is in a dependent relationship vis-à-vis the provider and the hospital, with the sick role legitimized by the physician.[20] In most instances, it is still the physician who serves as the gatekeeper of health care systems, although this is changing in some areas of primary care and in managed care systems where nurses perform a triage function. In other words, one does not have access to health care without a provider's sanction. The patients' rights movement seeks a new model for these relationships in which the traditional provider–patient relationship based on beneficence becomes more of a cooperative partnership in the attainment of health—a shared decision-making process.

Adequately informed consent is another mechanism for ensuring that the patient is a more active participant in dealing with the uncertainties of medical care and the lack of ready guarantees for specific patient outcomes. This requires that patients give up the illusion and expectation that physicians can cure all their medical problems. Chronic illness points to this reality as one must learn to live with whatever limitations are imposed.

The Bill of Rights is presented here in its entirety because it still serves as the basis for patient bills of rights established in hospitals, nursing homes, and other health care organizations. Patient bills of rights in hospitals generally incorporate patient responsibilities and obligations, such as keeping appointments, timely payment of bills, and consideration for other patients.

AMERICAN HOSPITAL ASSOCIATION STATEMENT ON A PATIENT'S BILL OF RIGHTS*

1. The patient has the right to considerate and respectful care.
2. The patient has the right to obtain from his physician complete current information concerning his diagnosis, treatment, and prognosis in terms the patient can be reasonably expected to understand. When it is not medically advisable to give such information to the patient, the information should be made available to an appropriate person in his behalf. He has the right to know by name the physician responsible for coordinating his care.
3. The patient has the right to receive from his physician information necessary to give informed consent prior to the start of any procedure and/or treatment. Except in emergencies, such information for informed consent should include but not necessarily be limited to the specific procedure and/or treatment, the medically significant risks involved, and the probable duration of incapacitation. Where medically significant alternatives for care or treatment exist, or when the patient requests information concerning medical alternatives, the patient has the right to such information. The patient also has the right to know the name of the person responsible for the procedures and/or treatment.
4. The patient has the right to refuse treatment to the extent permitted by law, and to be informed of the medical consequences of his action.
5. The patient has the right to every consideration of his privacy concerning his own medical care program. Case discussion, consultation, examination, and treatment are confidential and should be conducted discreetly. Those not directly involved in his care must have the permission of the patient to be present.
6. The patient has the right to expect that all communications and records pertaining to his care should be treated as confidential.
7. The patient has the right to expect that within its capacity a hospital must make reasonable response to the request of a patient for services. The hospital must provide evaluation, service and/or referral as indicated by the urgency of the case. When medically permissible, a patient may be transferred to another facility only after

he has received complete information and explanation concerning the needs for the alternatives to such a transfer. The institution to which the patient is to be transferred must first have accepted the patient for transfer.

8. The patient has the right to obtain information as to any relationship of his hospital to other health care and educational institutions insofar as his care is concerned. The patient has the right to obtain information as to the existence of any professional relationships among individuals, by name, who are treating him.

9. The patient has the right to be advised if the hospital proposes to engage in or perform human experimentation affecting his care or treatment. The patient has the right to refuse to participate in such research projects.

10. The patient has the right to expect reasonable continuity of care. He has the right to know in advance what appointment times and physicians are available and where. The patient has the right to expect that the hospital will provide a mechanism whereby he is informed by his physician or a delegate of the physician of the patient's continuing health care requirements following discharge.

11. The patient has the right to examine and receive an explanation of his bill regardless of source of payment.

12. The patient has the right to know what hospital rules and regulations apply to his conduct as a patient.

These proclaimed rights are legally unenforceable except in those states that have legislated the Patients' Bill of Rights and where they are already found in some hospital charters. W. Gaylin, a psychiatrist and cofounder of The Hastings Center, which studies our society's ethical problems, made the point that the AHA Patient's Bill of Rights reflects the paternalism practiced in the hospital setting and only gives back to patients the rights that hospitals have so long ignored.[21]

Even if many of these rights are legally unenforceable, they provide patients, families, and providers with knowledge of those specific rights that consumers might expect and demand as an expression of respect for the dignity of the individual. Annas reminds us that if rights are not exercised, they may be forgotten and violations of them may become routine.[22] This declaration of patient rights is even more important in today's health care environment, in which cost-containment efforts so often seem to be driving most organizational decision making, including patient care decisions.

Some states, such as Minnesota, have legislated the patient bill of rights and such advance directives as the so-called "living will," so that they do have legal standing as well as moral standing. The advance directive is an effort to further ensure patient rights to receive or refuse treatment and to direct treatment decisions if the patient is unable to do

---

*Reprinted with permission of the American Hospital Association, 840 North Lake Shore Drive, Chicago, Illinois 60611.

so. Another side of the patient rights coin is that even legally mandated rights must be enforced in today's complex and turbulent health care settings where the actual and potential threat of lawsuits is sometimes an overriding fear for health care providers. Legislation does serve one of the purposes that Macklin points to in her comments that "rights" language and the proclamation of those rights can be used to generate action and appropriate policy development by health care organizations that might not occur otherwise.

The reader may be wondering, "why all the discussion about legally enforceable rights?" Are there any rights and obligations that are granted for "humanitarian" or moral reasons based on one's membership in the human community? Talk about legal rights seems to reinforce Macklin's perception that the language of rights does not seem to help us much in dealing with specific ethical issues and dilemmas in health care. And, indeed, when attempting to honor patient rights, we must consider ethical principles such as respect for persons, avoiding or preventing harm while benefitting patients, and distributive justice.

Hospitals have created another mechanism for taking patient rights more seriously by employing patient representatives, that is, individuals who are skilled in patient relations. While these individuals do not necessarily serve as patient advocates, some do see their positions in this light. Most often, patient representatives deal with nonnursing and nonmedical matters related to patient comfort and convenience during hospitalization and are more accurately described as management's representative to patients. Annas argues that patient advocates *should* have medical care and treatment as their major concern. In that context, the advocate should have the following powers to be able to fulfill the duties of patient advocate: access to all the patient's hospital records, active participation in hospital committees monitoring quality of patient care, power to present patient complaints directly to the hospital administrator and the hospital's executive committee, access to all chiefs of service, access to patient support services, and the ability to delay discharges. Existing patient advocate systems do not generally follow this model.[23]

Several objections are raised to this role in the hospital setting: (1) that it interferes with current medical practice; (2) that patients' rights are already protected through informed consent and peer review; and (3) that it is only a "band-aid" approach to a fundamentally flawed health care delivery system. Another problem is that most patient representatives are employees of the hospital. When there are patient–hospital conflicts, the patient representative is accountable to the hospital rather than to the patient. Annas suggests that third party payers or health departments might provide the advocate's salary. He also agrees that the patient advocate's function is no panacea, but it does provide a mechanism for taking patient rights seriously, and this is necessary because the informed consent process does not ensure patient rights in health care bureaucracies where paternalistic practices still occur and vulnerable individuals feel intimidated.

FURTHER THOUGHTS FOR NURSING PRACTICE

Nurses and physicians often maintain that they serve as patient "advocates." What they mean when invoking the term is generally not made clear although it is commonly understood to mean identifying and following the patients' wishes. This meaning is hardly adequate for nurses, however, because the idea has the potential to make nurses a means to patient ends and to negate nurses' autonomy as moral beings.

Health and medical care providers are employed in hospitals and nursing homes in states where it is necessary to *legislate* patients' bills of rights. One might ask who, then, does advocate for patients and their rights when they are unable to do so in what is generally an intimidating environment or what Annas graphically describes as "a human rights wasteland."[24] Furthermore, the available technologies that are used to keep patients alive perpetuate the traditional medical ethic of doing everythirig possible for the individual patient but often are used without taking the patient's perspective into account. The patient's perspective may well differ from that of the provider; the patient may wish to refuse certain types of recommended treatments or use of all available technologies in an effort to cure when care is the more appropriate mode for that specific patient. It has also been pointed out that nurses cannot advocate for patients in the sense of ensuring their rights because nurses, as employees, are not accountable solely to patients even though this is a stance of the Code for Nurses. Nurses are accountable to numerous others, such as themselves, employers, and physicians.

Nurses must look at the specific ways in which they encourage or discourage patient or client autonomy, within the limits of safety and standards of nursing care, in hospitals, nursing homes, and other settings, such as the home or workplace. Nursing behavior that is appropriate for the comatose patient changes, or should change, dramatically when a conscious patient is being cared for and there is the need to ensure respect for patient autonomy. As patients expect or demand that their rights be honored in health care settings, what is nursing's response? Is the individual labeled as another "difficult" patient or family member? Kelly affirms that the nurse's direct responsibility is to explain nursing care and to provide health education, which is now spelled out in some state-legislated definitions of nursing so that health education is a legal as well as moral nursing obligation to patients.[25] This nursing obligation to assist patients in obtaining and deliberating about the information necessary to informed decision making holds tremendous implications. It is a key area for nurses who plan for continuity of care in the context of shorter hospitalizations for many patients and the reality that many procedures formerly done in the hospital are done on an outpatient basis. Such nursing obligations are critical when nurses are caring for terminally ill and dying patients and participating in or conducting patient care research.

Kelly points out that nurses as well as patients are taking risks if nurses choose to encourage and reinforce the exercise of patient rights with the possible risk of losing their jobs. As said before, if nurses choose to be more responsible and accountable to the patient, as supported in the Code for Nurses, there must be supportive environments for this kind of practice—that is, there must be a collegial nursing system. How long will ethical nursing practice be compromised by fear and by lack of formal colleague support? What are implications at the policy-making level for institutions that employ nurses if all nurses teach patients what they need to know about their chronic health problems in order to live with them if a physician does not want this done? What would happen to the image of nursing and to the health care structure if nurses did truly become patient advocates by creating an environment in which patients could make better-informed decisions about their health and in which patient goals and values would always be considered in decision making when patients were unable to do this for themselves? The responses to these questions by nurses, individually and collectively, affect patient care and nursing practice in profound ways. The ANA Code for Nurses and the ANA Standards for Nursing Practice support more ethical nursing practice and can be used to take positions on advocacy. Nurses could form a consensus and actively work to put into practice the principle of respect for patient and nurse autonomy and respect for patients and nurses as members of health care communities.

Hospital patients' and nursing home residents' bills of rights offer nurses, individually and collectively, opportunities to protect and to assist patients and residents in exercising their rights through participation in decisions affecting their care, to ensure that the patient's voice is heard when the patient is unable to participate, and to ensure that patients' wishes are heard with regard to any procedures, including nursing procedures. Nurses are in an even more critical position with regard to guaranteeing respect of patient rights in hospitals, given shorter stays and a continuing nursing shortage in critical patient care areas. Nurses have stated that such conditions put patient safety and welfare in jeopardy.

Mechanisms to assist nurses in an advocacy role include: learning to identify patient care situations in which ethical principles and values are at stake, participation on institution-wide and nursing ethics committees, initiating and conducting ethics rounds on patient care units, and incorporating identified ethical considerations in nursing decisions made with and for patients. GR Winslow, a professor of religion, argues that for nurses to serve successfully as patient advocates, there must be further clarification of the meaning of advocacy in nursing practice, review and revision of states' nurse practice acts, public education in order for patients and families to understand the advocacy role of nurses, an understanding by nurses of the difficulties and challenges surrounding the practice of patient advocacy, and preparation of nurses to deal with controversy surrounding advocacy for patients in complex bureaucratic structures.[26]

Fagin suggests that achievement and exercise of nurses' rights is a prerequisite to nurses helping patients achieve their rights.[27] Nursing's tradition and history have focused on responsibility and service of the nurse as a helping professional rather than autonomy and nurses' rights. Fagin sees nurses' rights emerging out of human rights and women's rights, since the majority of nurses are women. One's human rights ought to encompass the creation of situations that will enhance "humanness," for example, feelings of compassion, sympathy, and intelligence. Involved in women's rights are freedom of choice, equality, and respect for the individual person. This does not mean asking for special privileges but for the right to equal and full participation in such areas as decision making that affects one's practice, the right to the type of environment that allows for professional nursing practice and professional economic rewards, rights to a work environment that minimizes physical and emotional stresses, the right to set standards for excellence in nursing practice, and the right to participate in development of policy that affects nurses and nursing care. One can argue that it is the obligation of nursing to exercise such rights. Why? It is in order that nurses' rights not be permanently lost in depersonalized bureaucracies, where physicians provide direct care perceived by the public as valuable but where the direct care provided by nurses is often attributed to the physician's orders and is an unidentified aspect of hospital or institutional services, nurses as invisible providers. Direct billing for nursing services is one possible mechanism for changing this perception, with a challenge to maintain the caring in nursing care at the same time that care is treated as a commodity.

Assertion of rights for nurses in their practice is not an end in and of itself but is the means to improved services for patients and clients and more ethically adequate nursing practice. While the ANA Code for Nurses addresses itself primarily to nursing *obligations*, it also provides a framework for discussion of special *rights* of nurses derived from the special relationship of nursing to society as an essential service to those in need of nursing care and expertise, such as individuals who are critically ill and at-risk population groups.[28] Integral to the concept of nursing responsibilities and obligations is the authority or right to fulfill one's responsibilities as a professional person, that is, as a nurse in this instance. Responsibility without the corresponding right or authority to discharge one's professional obligations as a nurse leads to feelings of powerlessness and a sense of moral inadequacy in one's practice. The nurse's sense of integrity is in jeopardy under such circumstances, with profound implications for the individual nurse, for patient care, and for the nursing profession. Philosopher Nel Noddings expressed this idea powerfully in her comment: "There can be no greater evil, then, than this: that the moral autonomy of the one-caring be so shattered that she (or he) acts against her own commitment to care."[29]

Some would argue that nurses have no special rights. Generally, rights of health care professionals are considered as privileges that are carved out of patient or client rights. We argue that nurses do have special rights that can be considered as derivative from nursing responsibilities to clients. It is possible to argue that if nursing care is considered to be a societal necessity and right of those in need, then nurses have a corresponding responsibility *and* special right to provide nursing care to clients, care without which clients would suffer. While rights of individuals to nursing care are of great importance, they are not absolute in the sense of overriding all other considerations. For example, patients do not have a right to insist that nurses provide services that violate the bounds of acceptable practice or a nurse's own deeply held moral beliefs.

How do nurses' rights and obligations fit with situations where nurses question whether to accept or reject care of a particular client or group of clients? It can be argued that health care professionals have a duty to accept some personal risk of disease if in doing so another's life can be prolonged or their suffering decreased. This is even a societal expectation. At the same time, nurses are not morally required to put themselves at serious personal risk, though they (and others) have and may choose to do so. Nurses have the right to knowledge necessary to make informed decisions about provision of nursing care in such situations. Adequately informed decison making is essential for both clients and nurses and might be viewed as a fundamental human right. While putting one's self at serious personal risk can be understood as above and beyond what can be reasonably expected or required, nurses have an obligation never to abandon their patients. They should make arrangements for the client's necessary nursing care through individual *and* collective action if they choose not to provide the necessary care after careful thought and reflection.

Special nursing rights can also be derived from professional standards of nursing practice, the ANA Code for Nurses, and in the Nursing Services Section of the Joint Committee for the Accreditation of Hospitals (JCAH) *Accreditation Manual for Hospitals* (1982). It is up to nurses individually and collectively to work together in using these documents as support for changing inadequate or unsafe conditions of patient care in health care systems. Achievement of such nurses' rights could also help patients to exercise their rights, to meet obligations for their own health maintenance, and to reduce costs of care. This has been demonstrated. When nurses worked together to achieve an environment for professional practice at the Iowa Veterans Home in Marshalltown, Iowa, the residents became more active collectively in developing mechanisms for participating in decision making that affected their welfare.[30] While some of these activities may not be realistic in short-term acute care settings, nurses have an obligation and special rights to consider the consequences for the welfare of nurses and patients if such environments cannot be achieved in acute care settings. Primary nursing care and shared governance models are steps toward providing environments where patients may be heard and respected as individuals, promoting quality patient care, and demonstrating care for nurses and nursing practice as well.

Nurses can claim both obligations *and* special rights to ensure safe client care environments for the public where standards of practice and the Code for Nurses are explicitly used to guide nursing practice and caring. Achievement of more ethical nursing practice that ensures the integrity of nurses and the nursing care received by the public is another example of a responsibility and special right. These responsibilities and special rights of nurses require a new mindset, ethical reflection, decision making, and action, often political action. To talk about nurses' and patients' rights without acting to make them come alive is to surrender to passivity and further dependence on others. This is not a true vision of what professional nursing can and should be for both nurses and patients. Nurses can and do protect patient welfare at the bedside, in homes, and at policy-making levels of institutions and communities.

Issues of rights and obligations do not have to automatically remain in the realm of ethical dilemmas. Nurses can take preventive action to make decisions and take collective action to make patients' rights and nurses' special rights become realized rights by creating environments where patients' and nursings' values are a necessary part of the decision-making process.

REFERENCES

1. Summers J: Take patient rights seriously to improve patient care and to lower costs. *Health Care Manage Rev* 10:55–62, Fall 1985.
2. Report of American Nurses' Association Committee on Ethics to House of Delegates: *Enhancing Quality of Care Through Understanding Nurses' Responsibilities and Rights*. Kansas City, MO: American Nurses' Association; June 1986.
3. Jellinek M: Erosion of patient trust in large medical centers. *Hastings Cent Rep* 6:16–19, June 1976.

4. Bandman B: The human rights of patients, nurses, and other health professionals. In Bandman EL, Bandman B (eds): *Bioethics and Human Rights*. Boston: Little, Brown; 1978, pp 321–322.
5. Macklin R: Moral concerns and appeals to rights and duties. *Hastings Cent Rep* 6:32,34, October 1976.
6. Curran WJ: Lecture given in Human Rights and Health, Harvard School of Public Health, October 5, 1976.
7. Macklin: Moral concerns, p 37.
8. Ibid., p 31.
9. Gorovitz S, Jameton AL, Macklin R, et al (eds.): *Moral Problems in Medicine*. Englewood Cliffs, NJ: Prentice-Hall; 1976; pp 426–427.
10. Macklin: Moral concerns, p 32.
11. Ibid: pp 35–36.
12. President's Commission for the Study of Ethical Problems in Medicine and Biomedical and Behavioral Research: *Securing Access to Health Care*. Volume One: Report. U.S. Government Printing Office, March 1983, p. 20.
13. Callahan D: Health and society: Some ethical imperatives. *Daedalus* 106:30–32, Winter 1977.
14. Sade RM: Medical care as a right: A refutation. *N Engl J Med* 285:1288–1292, December 2, 1971.
15. Illich I: *Medical Nemesis: The Expropriation of Health*. Toronto: McClelland and Stewart; 1975.
16. Sparer EV: The legal right to health care. *Hastings Cent Rep* 6:39, October 1976.
17. President's Commission: *Securing Access to Health Care*, p 4.
18. Callahan D: *What Kind of Life?* New York: Simon & Schuster; 1989.
19. *Wilmington General Hospital v Manlove*, 54 Del 15, 174 A2d 135 (1961).
20. Bloom SW, Wilson RN: Patient–practitioner relationships. In Freeman HE, Levine S, Reeder LG (eds): *Handbook of Medical Sociology*, 2nd ed. Englewood Cliffs, NJ: Prentice-Hall; 1972; pp 315–332.
21. Gaylin W: The patients' bill of rights. *Saturday Rev Sci* 1:22, March 1973. Editorial.
22. Annas GJ: *The Rights of Hospital Patients: The Basic ACLU Guide to a Hospital Patient's Rights*. New York: Avon; 1975. Preface.
23. Annas GJ: *Judging Medicine*. Clifton, NJ: Humana; 1988, p 22.
24. Ibid. p 4.
25. Kelly LY: The patient's right to know. *Nurs Outlook* 24:27, January 1976.
26. Winslow GR: From loyalty to Advocacy: A new metaphor for nursing. *Hastings Cent Rep* 14:38–39, June 1984.
27. Fagin CM: Nurses' rights. *Am J Nurs* 75:82–85, January 1975.
28. Report of American Nurses' Association Committee on Ethics: *Enhancing Quality of Care*.
29. Noddings N: *Caring: A Feminine Approach to Ethics and Moral Education*. Berkeley: University of California Press; 1984, p 115.
30. Maas J, Jacox AK: *Guidelines for Nurse Autonomy/Patient Welfare*. New York: Appleton-Century-Crofts; 1977, p 149.

CHAPTER 7

Informed Consent

ETHICAL PRINCIPLES OF INFORMED CONSENT

Informed consent is grounded in the ethical principle of autonomy when the patient speaks for himself or herself. Generally speaking, this means in bioethics that individuals have the right to information and, on the basis of this input, the right to agree or to refuse to participate in research or to undergo the treatment being proposed. Autonomy means that persons have the right to determine their course of action on the basis of a plan that they have developed for themselves. This does not mean that no limits on autonomy exist. Some individuals, because of their physical or mental conditions, have diminished autonomy. Others, such as institutionalized populations, also tend to have less autonomy in their daily lives because of their social situation. In addition, autonomy does not mean that individuals can do anything they want. The reasons people have for their autonomous actions are their own reasons, but they must be principled and not arbitrary reasons.[1]

When patients make decisions based on necessary and clear information, they are acting as autonomous agents. From an ethical perspective, health professionals have the obligation to respect their decisions, even in those situations where they disagree with the patient. There are complex exceptions to these general situations, such as when parents decide on a course of action for their child that is harmful and might even lead to death. Another exception can be found in emergency situations where the health professionals have the primary obligation to treat.

Informed consent also acts to safeguard patients by preventing harm being done to them. This involves the ethical principle of nonmaleficence, or the responsibility to do no harm. It is possible that patients may choose to be involved in research that includes substantial risk for them. In these cases, patients exercise their autonomy by choosing a potentially greater risk than might be chosen for them by someone else. Because they decide for themselves, with an understanding of what is involved, harm is not done and autonomous actions occur.

In addition to the ethical principles of autonomy and nonmalefi-cence, informed consent can also serve to protect all of society by en-couraging self-scrutiny among health professionals and researchers and by involving the public in these matters.[2] This is the ethical principle of utility. It is useful in a democratic society to have informed, involved people.

It is important to realize that although several ethical principles support informed consent, the major and most central justification for it is the principle of autonomy. As Beauchamp and Childress have said, "There is a moral duty to seek a valid consent *because* the consenting party is an autonomous person, with all the entitlements that status confers."[3] This autonomous person status is the reason we obtain in-formed consent even when there is no risk to the patient or research subject and when no immediate social utility occurs.

People can give informed consent only if they have sufficient infor-mation on which to base a decision. An ethical principle girding the giving of information is veracity, or truth telling. Trust in professional relations with clients and patients comes in part from veracity. The ethical question is when, if ever, it is ethically justified to withhold the truth as we know it from the patient.

RESEARCH AND INFORMED CONSENT

Any discussion of informed consent must be placed within the larger context of the moral justification for conducting research using human subjects. In much, if not most, biomedical research with human sub-jects, we usually assume that previous trials have been conducted on animals and that there has been careful assessment of predictable risks in comparison with foreseeable benefits. Although the moral issues of using animals in research to better the human condition are worthy of our close attention, they remain outside the present discussion.[4,5]

In order to proceed with a discussion of why and whether we should conduct research using human subjects, some definitions will be helpful. Therapy refers to a class of activity intended to benefit an individual or member of a group. The person giving therapy has the in-tention of benefiting the recipient of the activity. Research, on the other hand, refers to scientific activity intended to contribute to the general knowledge in a field. Two subtypes of research can be identified. First, scientists conduct therapeutic research mainly for the benefit of the subject while also gaining knowledge. For example, the giving of a new drug to a cancer patient can be basically for therapeutic purposes while at the same time it can be a trial test for the drug. Second, scientists also engage in nontherapeutic research using human subjects to gain new knowledge. An example is an experiment that deliberately introduces change into a given situation and then measures and compares the respective effects on the control group and the experimental group. The control group does not usually benefit in any therapeutic way from the research. The motivation to participate of those in the control group is not therapeutic benefit but for the rewards from or of advancement of science.

Conducting research using human subjects can be morally justified on the basis of the ethics of good consequences. We all derive social benefits from research, whether that benefit is immediately therapeutic to us personally or whether it affects us indirectly by affecting resources. Eventually a procedure or a drug, after being tested on nonhumans, must be tested on some humans so that the knowledge gained can be used for the larger social good. Furthermore, serious harm would develop from not conducting research using human subjects, since scientific advances would be greatly limited. When you think about it, most of the health care measures, both preventive and curative, that we now take for granted were once experimental and involved human subjects in their development. We can morally justify using human subjects by arguing from a utilitarian position that the practice produces good consequences for the greater number of people.

Using the concept of justice, one can also develop a nonconsequential argument to support and morally justify nontherapeutic research. We, as a society, benefit from the risks that others have taken in previous experiments; therefore, is it just for us to reap these benefits without reciprocal action? The fact that in biomedical research a time arrives when only human subjects can provide the data needed must neither overshadow nor obscure the ethical dilemmas involved.

Morally justifying the use of humans in experimentation does not eliminate all of the possible ethical dilemmas that can confront the researcher once such research gets under way. Such considerations as freedom of choice and coercion, rights of the individual and needs of society, the meaning of "the good," and the problem of uncertainty in determining the risk–benefit ratio represent some of the more obvious dimensions of these ethical dilemmas.

Research experimentation using humans as subjects can be traced back to the beginning of recorded history. This early research, mainly conducted in an unsystematic fashion within the clinical practice context, lead to instances of patients receiving treatments whose value had not been established by controlled, well-designed clinical investigation. There have also been reported many instances of researchers and health care professionals, including nurses, submitting themselves as subjects in research projects.

Few questions arose over the years with regard to these practices, since it was assumed that the individuals being used for research purposes also benefited as the recipients of the knowledge gained in these

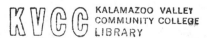

experimentations. Although the late 19th century saw an acceleration in the systematic use of human subjects for research purposes, this activity did not lead to an exploration of the need for safeguards protecting these individuals. One notable exception can be found in Bernard's 1865 publication, in which he demonstrated the need for research using human subjects and began to develop rules of ethical conduct to govern such an enterprise.[6]

Along with medicine, the law gave little attention to the rights of human subjects in experimentation. In the mid 1930s, the Michigan Supreme Court stated that experimentation, although important and necessary, must be undertaken with the knowledge and consent of the patient or someone responsible for him and such procedures must not vary too radically from accepted practice.[7] This broad generalization that the Court used to distinguish between rash experimentation with humans and systematic and ethical scientific research practice did not anticipate the grave concerns that arose in a few years from the Nuremberg disclosures. The atrocities perpetrated by German physicians in the name of clinical research during the Third Reich disturbed many scientists, who then wanted ethical standards established on a world-wide basis to protect human subjects.

REGULATIONS AND HUMAN SUBJECTS

The Nazi experiments, so far outside the limits of what anyone would consider accepted medical and research practice, tended to be viewed by some as a terrible and tragic moment in history but separate from the general problem of protection for research subjects. Such a view obscured the fact that in principle, although perhaps not in the same magnitude, many similar moral issues had characterized research since the beginning of experimentation. The Military Tribunal that tried the Nazi physicians formulated a code of ethics that has profoundly shaped the ethos of the experimental aspects of post-World War II biomedical research. Some excerpts from the code will illustrate the general nature of this document. The code states that voluntary consent of the human subject is absolutely essential and that the duty and responsibility for ascertaining the quality of the consent rests upon each individual who initiates, directs, or engages in the experiment. This personal duty and responsibility may not be delegated to another with impunity. The code also says that the experiment should be such as to yield fruitful results for the good of society unprocurable by other methods or means of study and not trivial or unnecessary in nature. Furthermore, the degree of risk to be taken should never exceed that determined by the humanitarian importance of the problem to be solved by the experiment. During the course of the experiment, the human subject should be at liberty to end his participation in the experiment if he reaches the physical or mental state where continuation seems to him to be impossible. In addition, the scientist must be prepared to terminate the experiment at any stage if he believes that a continuation of the experiment is likely to result in injury, disability, or death for the experiment's subject.

The promulgation of other codes of ethics, such as the World Medical Association Helsinki Declaration of 1964, the American Medical Association Ethical Guidelines for Clinical Investigation of 1966, the American Nurses' Association Human Rights Guidelines for Nurses in Clinical and Other Research of 1975, focused attention not only on the ethical dilemmas inherent in research activities but also on the limitation of codes. Succinctly worded and devoid of commentary, codes, although useful as general guidelines, cannot cover every possible eventuality and thus remain limited and subject to interpretation. These codes of ethics made it clear, however, that the professions recognized that self-regulation by investigators could not be relied on solely to safeguard the rights of human subjects in experiments. This realization, coupled with the growing awareness of the limitations of codes, led to the development of procedures to apply the general moral principles contained in the codes. The procedures took the form of formal evaluation of research projects by institutional review committees. In 1953, the National Institutes of Health developed procedures to regulate research conducted at its clinical center.[8] In 1971, the Department of Health, Education, and Welfare formulated its policy for the protection of human subjects, and at present these policies vest basic responsibility for the protection of human subjects in institutional review committees.[9] Because of the prominent role that the federal government has in funding biomedical research, over 700 institutions have established committees to review research protocols. These committees are called Institutional Review Boards (IRB). Such institutional committees in hospitals, medical centers, and other such facilities around the country are in charge of initial reviews of all research proposals and periodic re-review in order to ascertain that each researcher has outlined the risks and benefits and that the subjects have given their informed consent to participate in the study. Essentially, the IRB must determine that the rights and welfare of the subjects are protected, that the risks to an individual are outweighed by the potential benefits to him and society, and that informed consent will be obtained by adequate and appropriate methods. These governmental review standards, although worded in general terms, do detail the basic elements of informed consent, thereby drawing attention to its importance. Such standards should assist the scientific community in preventing future abuses like those in several of the more dramatic cases from the past: the cancer immunology experimentation at the Jewish Chronic Disease Hospital in New York, the hepatitis experiment on mentally retarded children institutionalized at Willowbrook, and the

Tuskegee syphilis study on Southern blacks.[10-12] These studies and others that received less media coverage show the extent to which the scientific merits of research can be overshadowed when the basic ethical principles pertaining to human dignity and human life of experimental subjects are violated.

The IRBs review research protocols at the local level, whereas the National Commission for the Protection of Human Subjects of Biomedical and Behavioral Research, an interdisciplinary group established in 1974 to advise the then Department of Health, Education, and Welfare (HEW), investigate the ethical principles of human experimentation, and develop guidelines for it on the national level. The Commission has published a number of important books that developed from its work. One such book addresses ethical issues surrounding informed consent.[13] The establishment of these commissions and councils and the development of guidelines and regulations are viewed by some professionals as onerous and even dangerous, because these activities may interfere with scientific advancement. Others, however, believe we require even more social control in these matters. They do not believe the present devices, including informed consent, protect human subjects enough from the ever-present potential for abuse.

INFORMED CONSENT

The scientist has the ethical obligation to provide disclosure of information that includes the proclamation of benefits, the warning of risks, and the discussion of quandaries in order to obtain consent from the potential research subject. This consent must be based on the subject's understanding of the information to the greatest extent possible in order for him to be considered properly informed.

The concept of informed consent grew from the malpractice litigation of the 1950s such as *Canterbury v Spence*, mentioned in Chapter 1, in which a young man became paralyzed after surgery and a fall. More specifically, it arose from legal cases in which the patient's attorney had difficulty proving a physician's negligence when the usual community standards of medical practice were used for comparison. The informed consent approach shifted the legal claim from a charge of negligence to one of battery, because the patient would not have consented to the procedure had he known of the possible risk. Since the doctor had not completely informed that patient as to these possible risks and alternatives, the patient had not given his informed consent. Without effective consent, the physician had treated or operated upon the patient in an unlawful manner. This use of informed consent theory helped the patient's lawyer in these types of cases, because other doctors did not have to testify as to community standards. Later, however, the courts determined that the requirement of informed consent would be measured by the community standards of medical practitioners. The concept of informed consent had by that time gained acceptance both in medical practice procedures and in research experimentation.

Two early studies that have become classics, published ten years apart, provide some insights into the ethical dilemmas involved in informed consent. In 1966, Beecher maintained that codes of ethics made the bland assumption that meaningful or informed consent was available for the asking, whereas in reality this very often was not the case.[14] Although he conceded that consent in the fullest sense may not be obtainable, he said that it remains a goal toward which every researcher must nevertheless strive. With this in mind, he reviewed 50 studies in which he found only two mentions of informed consent; 12 studies seemed unethical, and generally his data suggested widespread ethical issues, especially with regard to informed consent. Following the position of the British Medical Research Council, Beecher said that not only should all investigations be conducted in an ethical manner, but in the publications it should also be made unmistakably clear that the proprieties have been observed. He believed that journals have a moral obligation not to publish unethical research, even when those studies present very valuable data. Such a policy would discourage unethical experimentation. Beecher concluded by pointing out that the ethical approach has two important components, informed consent and the presence of an intelligent, informed, conscientious, compassionate, and responsible investigator. The other study, by Barber, published in 1976, made note of the fact that in the previous decade we had increasingly perceived a social problem in the abuse of human subjects in medical experimentation.[15] Two major reasons have led to this general recognition that experimentation with humans is a subject for concern: the increased power, scope, and funding of biomedical research and changes in values that have increased the emphasis on equality, participation, and the challenging of arbitrary authority. Barber and his colleagues conducted a national survey in which they found that whereas the majority of the investigators were what they called "strict" with regard to balancing risks against benefits, a significant minority were "permissive," or more willing to accept an unsatisfactory risk–benefit ratio. In light of the fact that most institutions and the federal government now require that the human subject in an experiment or his guardian understand that some treatment is being withheld or something is being done for reasons other than immediate therapy, and the fact that the subject or his guardian must be informed of any risks and must give consent voluntarily, Barber produced some interesting data. With regard to the issue of informed consent, these data again revealed a minority with "permissive" views and practices, although that minority was smaller than it was for an unfavorable risk–benefit ratio. These data raise the question of how it happens that the treatment of human subjects is sometimes less than ethical, even in some of the most respected university hospitals. Barber answered this question by saying that these abuses can be traced to defects in the training of researchers, to defects in the screening and monitoring of research by review committees, and to a fundamental tension between investigation and therapy.

In another early study, Gray interviewed 51 women who were, or had just been, subjects in another study to determine the effects of a new labor-inducing drug. His findings indicated that although all 51 women signed a consent form, 20 of them learned only from Gray's interview that they were research subjects. Of this group of 20, most of them did not understand that there might be hazards, that they would be subjected to special procedures, or that they were not required to participate in the study. Indeed, four of the women made it clear that they would not have participated had they understood and realized that they had a choice.[16]

For most authorities on the matter, the core of the informed consent process from the beginning of the discussion was the balancing of risk to the human subject against possible benefits to him and society. However, Jonas voiced resistance to this "merely utilitarian view." He raised the issue of the peculiarity of human experimentation quite independent of the question of possible injury to the subject. According to him, the wrong involved with making a person an experimental subject is not so much that we make him thereby a means to an end, since that happens in social contexts of all kinds, but that we make him a thing. He accused us of reducing the person in human experimentation to a passive thing or token, or a "sample" merely to be acted on.[17] This penetrating argument can help researchers to structure the ethical issues in their deliberations of means and ends, the individual good and the common good, and the private and the public welfare, all of which must be considered in informed consent.

Ideally, informed consent can be thought of as a collaborative endeavor involving truth telling on the part of the researcher and free choice on the part of the subject within a context of some degree of uncertainty. If we already knew all the possible risks and benefits of a given procedure or drug, we would not need to undertake the research. In determining the most accurate risk–benefit ratio, we need a thoughtful, humane, and best-educated opinion. It may prove easier to detail these possibilities more adequately in research that has been tested on nonhuman subjects. It also may be more difficult to ascertain the psychological impact or risks in all research. In addition, social science research may present special problems, since prior research on animals in most cases is inappropriate and impossible, and the possible psychological trauma experienced by human subjects sometimes remains underestimated and often unknown.

The Helsinki Declaration says that research involving human subjects cannot legitimately be carried out unless the importance of the objective is in proportion to the inherent risk to the subject. Such inherent risks may be easier to measure and weigh in the risk–benefit calculus with biomedical research than with research focused on psychological or social aspects. Nevertheless, the Helsinki Declaration does say that every precaution should be taken to minimize the impact of the study on the subject's physical and mental integrity and on the personality of the subject.

It has been documented that the social sciences differ from the natural sciences in some fundamental ways. Although uncertainty exists in the natural sciences, the difficulty in observing and analyzing social reality presents other very complex social science problems. The objects of social science research are living conditions, institutions, or human attitudes that combine changeability and rigidity in an unstable and, to some extent, an inscrutable pattern. Some social scientists have attempted to emulate the methods of natural sciences and this has at times led to a dangerous superficiality in approach. Such an analysis, regarded as strict or rigorous by natural science standards, may in social science research be lacking in both logical consistency and adequate reflection of reality.

In the research projects of both natural science and social science, the importance of the research also becomes a factor. Some research may have minimum risk but also minimum benefits to the subject and society. Should such research be done? How could we either support it or not on moral grounds? If such research includes inconveniences rather than risks to the human subjects, are there ethical considerations nonetheless? A more serious problem arises in the instance in which there is possible risk but minimum benefit involved in the study. In some research, the procedure is so intrusive that the possible risks become more obvious, whereas when the procedures are less intrusive, the possible risks may be overlooked. In each experimental situation, such dimensions of the risk–benefit ratio need reviewing with the potential human subject before an informed consent is obtained.

In all research, the possible dilemma arises as to the extent of the disclosure necessary to obtain a truly informed consent. In the past, when a patient engaged a physician or entered a hospital, these actions themselves often served as a blanket consent to such treatment as the physician or hospital staff, in the exercise of their professional judgment, deemed proper. Now the extent and the content of the disclosure for treatment purposes has expanded, taking into account the patient's rights and the professional's obligations.

The similar problem in research, noted over 35 years ago, results from the combination of helplessness, lack of technical competence, and the emotional disturbance experienced in the sick role that make the patient a peculiarly vulnerable object for exploration.[18] While this view of the totally passive and helpless patient as put forth by the sociologist Parsons has raised questions, it does acknowledge an uneven balance in information and power between the person obtaining informed consent and the person giving it. This, combined with the argument that patients do not want to know or cannot understand, has made informed consent a necessity. Patients not only have the right to know and to make decisions, but as one study found, the majority of them want to know what possible complications may be expected from any given procedure. This study concluded that the concern that informing the patient of possible complications will result in his refusal of the procedure is now outmoded.[19]

In these earlier discussions of informed consent, Baumrind made one of the more profound observations in discussing the issue of human experimentation. She maintained that subjects are less adversely affected by physical pain or psychological stress than by experiences that result in loss of trust in themselves and the investigators and, by extension, in the meaningfulness of life itself. The researcher violates the fundamental moral principles of reciprocity and justice when he, using his position of trust, acts to deceive or degrade those whose extension of trust has been granted on the basis of a contrary role expectation. He behaves unjustly when he uses naive (trusting) subjects and then exploits their naivete, no matter if the direct resulting harm is small. The harm becomes cumulative both to the individual and to society.[20] This ethical position has had an impact on studies that in the past relied on deception to obtain their findings. Studies undertaken by Milgram, Hofling et al, Humphrey, and Rosenhan provide but a few examples of such research.[21-24] None of these studies, with publication dates ranging from 1965 to 1973, would today be approved by an IRB. Some argue that they are important studies and give us knowledge and insights that we would not otherwise have. While this may be true, our ethics has developed in obtaining informed consent to safeguard the human subject. Research that relies on deception makes that obligation difficult to meet. Alison Lurie pushed the limits of deception in research and the undercover role of the scientist in her novel about two academic research sociologists.[25] Regardless of the importance of the findings in these and other such studies, a serious ethical dilemma underlies the entire research structure. To rely on deception means that the researcher totally violates the ethical principle of truth-telling and dupes a subject who cannot give his informed consent in a situation in which he has not been told the real nature of the research or indeed that he is participating in research at all. The question is usually raised as to whether this means that some research cannot or should not be performed. Yes, it does possibly mean just that. Another question raised relates to the problem of biasing the research by giving the subject too much detail. In this case, at least two solutions to the issue of informed consent exist. First, it may be possible to redesign the research so that disclosure will not bias the study. Second, it may be possible to tell the subject some details and also discuss the fact that to go into more details would make the research findings less reliable. The latter solution has possible problems, since, although the subject knows information is being withheld, he is not aware of the nature of the information.

As imperfect as it may be, the written informed consent procedure does accord the patient the status of a person, not an experimental animal, and provides a degree of assurance that he is being considered as an end and not merely as a means. Respect for human dignity and individuality is historically linked with a freedom of scientific inquiry that is equally precious to modern liberalism. Like most norms, the basic principles of human experimentation have been formulated on such an abstract level that they provide only general guides to actual behavior. Insofar as every treatment procedure and every involvement in research carry with them potential risk, it must be the patient or his guardian who has the right to decide not only whether to participate but also what factors are or are not relevant to his consent. This ethical position draws the line at full disclosure in most, if not all, instances, but it also allows room for judgments to be made in the individual, concrete situation.[26] Several authors have identified potential problems in the process of informed consent.[27-30] One study has concluded that consent forms always may have been too difficult for typical volunteers to comprehend. In examining the effects of federal regulations on the readability and length of consent forms used in medical research from 1975 through 1982, the researchers found that the difficulty levels may have increased since 1975.[31] In another study it was found that awareness and understanding are greater if the investigators themselves explain the research to the patient and do not leave this responsibility to others. It also helps the consent process if the investigators ask for feedback from patients to ascertain how much they understand and whether more information needs to be given.[32] In the long run, all the regulations, reviews, and informed consent forms will serve a limited function unless the clinician and researcher bring their ethical reasoning and integrity to bear on these complex issues.

INFORMED CONSENT AND SELECTED HUMAN SUBJECTS

The concept of informed consent rests on the assumption that the researcher will adequately inform the potential research subject, in language he can understand, so that the individual or his guardian will in fact understand the risks and benefits and will be in a position either to agree to participate or to refuse to do so without negatively affecting his relationship with the researcher or the institution providing the service. Competent people have the right to decide whether to accept or reject proposed treatment and being in a research protocol. The concept of competence, simply put, means that the patient has the ability to communicate choices, can understand relevant information, can appreciate the situation and its consequences, and can manipulate information rationally.[33] Certain groups present special ethical problems and raise questions regarding the adequacy of informed consent. Research using students, prisoners, minors, the mentally ill, the mentally retarded, the elderly, especially those in an institution, and fetuses can and do raise many ethical dilemmas.

The problem of restricted choice can arise in a number of situations ranging from research with students to that with prisoners and other institutionalized persons. For example, when the instructor in a classroom asks the students to volunteer for research purposes, there exists at least the implied threat of loss of affection and possibly poorer academic grades if the student does not volunteer. This becomes a situation of restricted choice for the student, with ethical dilemmas involved. Previously some institutions granted students credit for participating in research. This procedure raised the issue of infringement of the rights of those who did not volunteer or were not chosen after volunteering.

A more serious ethical dilemma can occur in research using prisoners as human subjects. During the 1970s, a number of individuals and groups voiced concern about using prisoners in human experimentation.[34-38] These concerns centered on a number of topics, including behavioral research, behavior control, drug tests, operant conditioning, psychosurgery, and castration, but the underlying ethical dilemma is: to what extent can prisoners exercise freedom of choice in giving consent or refusing it? The issues of restrictive choice and possible coercion have been weighed against the benefits to the individual prisoner, usually remuneration and better living conditions for research subjects, occasionally reduced sentences, benefits to society, and the obligations, if any, that the prisoner has to society. Many people concerned with this area of human experimentation believe that it may not be possible to overcome the serious ethical dilemmas. The fundamental ethical concepts embodied in the informed consent process can easily be violated in these circumstances.

A similar situation arises with the committed mentally ill patient, and the same ethical concerns may lead to the conclusion that informed consent is not a possibility. With voluntary patients in institutions, informed consent may be an adequate safeguard because of their legal status; however, that status can change and their choices can become restricted. Moreover, in either case, the patient's mental status caused by his illness or by drugs and his ability to give consent must be viewed as the basis for a potential ethical dilemma. Recent laws in some states have addressed the informed consent issue for both involuntary and voluntary patients with regard to the right to refuse drugs. However, the question has been raised as to whether such legislation as the Mental Health Act of 1983 really provides a useful safeguard for the protection of the psychiatric patient's civil rights.[39]

With the mentally retarded, the problems are mental status; being institutionalized and dependent; and, who speaks for and safeguards the rights of the individual being asked to serve as a human subject. If someone else consents for him to act as a subject, then that person must be informed and give consent with the best interest of the potential subject as the grounds for his actions. One can attempt to evaluate such action by asking what decision any reasonable person would make under these particular circumstances. Most likely, the characteristics of the ideal observer would be helpful in making the decision. Having all the information available, understanding potential consequences, coupled with the ability to visualize the experience as if it were happening to him (the observer), but also having the ability to be impartial, this observer ideally can make the best morally based decision. This observer represents an ideal, and not necessarily a reality, in any given individual; however, such characteristics may be found among the individuals in a small group as they discuss risks and direct or indirect benefit, or the lack of them, to the subject of the proposed research project.

Some doubts can be raised about the moral motivation of some parents in giving consent for their retarded institutionalized child to be part of a research study. This does not mean that all such parents are morally suspect, but a possible conflict of interest does exist in the situation. The child may possibly have been institutionalized because his parents reject him. In such a case, conflict of interest looms larger than in a situation where the child has been placed in an institution because he cannot be physically managed at home or elsewhere.

The staff members who conduct research with the mentally retarded in such an institution may have more of a conflict than some other researchers. Any research with the mentally retarded in any setting raises conflict of interest and other ethical dilemmas. A modified version of Rawls' publicity concept provides one mechanism for dealing with this situation. A group such as a ward unit group or a research review committee can examine the moral dimensions in a research protocol and determine whether the individuals being sought as human subjects should participate in the research and, if so, on what grounds, taking into account their rights as they would be exercised in a situation of choice.

Some of the same issues come into play in research with minors.[40-44] An unwritten rule in many hospitals says that a child of 7 or older can and should give his own informed consent, whereas a younger child has not developed moral reasoning, and it falls to his parent or guardian to give consent. One of the most serious questions with any group—and especially vulnerable ones, including well children—involves research that is nontherapeutic or nonbeneficial to the subject. On what ethical grounds should research be conducted using either well children or mentally ill or retarded children where risks must be weighed against benefits? For normal children, the benefits will be neither direct nor immediate in any tangible way. The questions become: Should physically well, normal children ever be human subjects? If so, on what moral grounds? Should mentally ill or retarded children participate in any research, and, if so, should it only be research that can potentially benefit them directly? If other research is to be permitted, on what moral grounds would these children become human subjects and who will speak for them in the informed consent procedure?

One area that has aroused much debate, that of fetal research, has also raised the issue of possible medical benefits gained as measured against the possible ethical costs of such research to society.[45-58] Some of this impassioned debate surrounding fetal research is tied to the different moral positions that people have taken on abortion. A discussion of the rights of the fetus can be found in Chapter 8.

The elderly, and particularly those in institutions such as nursing homes, represent another vulnerable group in the human subjects controversy. Many of the same issues mentioned above also arise with this group. And as with some of the other groups, we tend to have negative attitudes toward the elderly that may blur some of the ethical considerations.[59-61]

One researcher, in writing about the inequitable allocation of research risks, makes the point that new knowledge designed to benefit all society must not be gained at the expense of any individual or any segment of society. To this end he would restrict experimentation to those research projects directly concerned with issues of the group of individuals used or research that has higher than average probability of benefiting the specific category of persons or would lead to such knowledge as could be expected to reduce the need for hospitalization or confinement.[62]

With all potential subjects for research projects, and certainly with these special problem groups, many ethical dilemmas emerge. Although some think that the goal of having human subjects spontaneously volunteer rather than being conscripted cannot be achieved, nevertheless, most believe that efforts to promote educated, informed consent are in order. This effort to educate and inform should reach everyone, including these groups and others, such as the poor, who depend more on public facilities, where probably more training of health care personnel and more research occurs than in the private sector of the health care delivery system.

RISKS AND COMPENSATION

The individual's right to refuse to participate in research must be balanced against his obligations to society, the extent to which it will benefit him or others, and the potential risk involved. One 1976 report from the HEW, in an attempt to determine how many persons may be harmed by their participation in federally funded medical research, obtained data from 331 telephone interviews with investigators who conducted research in the preceding three years. A total of 133,000 human subjects participated in these studies. About half of the investigators reported that they did nontherapeutic research not expected to benefit study participants. Of about 93,000 subjects who participated in this nontherapeutic research, 0.8 percent were reported injured as a result of their participation. The authors concluded that this injury rate equals the annual rate of accidental injuries in this country that occur through ordinary living. Therefore, the risks of participation in nontherapeutic research may be no greater than those of everyday life. Of the 39,000 or so individuals who participated in therapeutic research in which there were treatments that could be expected to benefit the participants involved, 10.8 percent were reported as being injured in some way. Again, however, this rate equals that experienced as a result of ordinary treatment outside the research setting.

The issue of compensation for injured research subjects has received attention both from the law and from ethicists. Early in this discussion, the ethicist James Childress developed a detailed moral argument to use in thinking through the ethical dilemmas of this issue.[63] He considers the basis, scope, and limits of society's obligations to compensate injured research subjects within the framework of justice. Reparative justice, rendering each person his or her due, focuses on the fault of one party for an injury to another party, and the party causing the injury is blameworthy and held liable for it. On the other hand, compensatory justice is giving a person his or her due by taking account of a previous state of affairs and attempting to restore a "fallen" individual or group to it. Restoration can rarely be literal, and therefore it most often requires a monetary substitute. According to Childress, compensatory justice is a concrete application of the principle of fairness in the imposition of risks for the benefit of society. From this moral argument, only briefly touched upon here, he draws the conclusion that informed consent does not constitute a waiver of claims for compensation.

Informed consent implies joint adventure in a common cause, a partnership between subject and investigator, or a process of coinvestigation. It is the propensity to overreach this joint adventure, even in a good cause, that makes consent necessary. This agreement however, cannot substitute for the wisdom and moral integrity of the researcher.

INFORMED CONSENT AND TREATMENT

In treatment we assume that patients benefit directly, whereas in research they may or may not benefit directly in return for participation. The elements of informed consent that operate in research situations are valid in treatment situations as well. Patients should not receive treatment except in emergencies until they have given consent that is informed. Although there are many issues in informed consent and treatment, this discussion is limited to two issues: withholding information and the patients' comprehension of the information given.

Rarely is good news withheld. Sometimes bad news, such as the diagnosis of cancer or something as bad, is withheld from the patient. If the patient is a competent adult who is capable of acting autonomously, the decision to withhold information from him or her violates the ethical principle of veracity and renders the patient less than autonomous. The decision to withhold information often is derived from the ethical principle of nonmaleficence, or the obligation to do no harm. The reasoning is as follows: The patient is very ill and is suffering. We should not further burden him or her with knowledge of the seriousness of the diagnosis. Such good intentions in the name of doing no harm result in curtailment of the patient's autonomy and create a deceitful situation for all those around the patient. The truth can be cruel, and the way we inform patients must take this into account. Great sensitivity and adequate emotional support for the patient are required. When this sort of ethical dilemma arises, it needs to be reasoned through and the ethical principles weighed to determine which is to be followed and which is to be violated, since in these situations, both cannot be followed. How this is to be accomplished must then be worked out.

Available data can assist in a general way in reaching a solution to this ethical dilemma. Since the mid-1940s the vast majority of articles on whether to tell the patient the truth supply the ethical justification for telling, even when the news is considered to be bad.[64-72] In addition, research conducted over the past 40 years asking patients and potential patients if they want to be told their diagnosis, even if it is bad news, indicates that most people do want to have this information.[73-79] One paper does maintain that under certain conditions the surrender of decision making by the patient, in the acceptance of a paternalistic relationship, is morally justifiable and, by the very nature of a paternalistic physician–patient relationship, a valid informed consent is seldom if ever realizable and is, for the most part, of no concern to the patient.[80]

A major criticism of informed consent is that patients cannot understand the complex information they need to be able to give informed consent. Poor distribution of power and information exists. Informed consent is not a perfect tool, but with more attention to the ethics underlying it and a focus on pragmatic aspects of the process, the patient should be better able to participate in the decision making involved in his treatment and care.

INFORMED CONSENT AND NURSING

In the most fundamental sense, the moral principle underlying informed consent was addressed by Kant when he said that we ought to treat mankind as an end and never merely as a means.[81] But, as has been noted, it sounds strange to speak of persons as ends, even though the Kantian formula is familiar to us. As has been implied so far in this chapter, we regard persons as valuable in themselves, not for what we can get out of them but because they are persons. To say that something—in this case, a person—is valuable in itself does not exclude the possibility that it is also valuable as a means. Many of our problems arise when we consider persons *merely* as a means. One of the most detailed commentaries on the principle of respect for persons says that we ought to treat people as valuable in themselves and not only as useful instruments.[82]

Over the years, a number of comments have been made about ethical issues or dilemmas and human rights as related to nursing practice and research.[83-85] This discussion includes selected aspects of informed consent in research and treatment and the nurse's obligations. Abdellah, in a paper based on a presentation at the 1967 National League for Nursing Convention, noted that as nursing research focused more on clinical problems, the legal and ethical aspects would become more apparent. Although clinical nursing research may differ from medical research in the extent and kind of risk to patients, in both disciplines many similar problems exist regarding conduct of research. At that time, according to Abdellah, much clinical nursing research used the behavioral science methods, such as interviews, questionnaires, and observations, to obtain data. There were a number of ethical issues, including the right to privacy or to withhold information.[86] It is helpful to know that just two years before, in June 1965, the United States Supreme Court had given an opinion to the case of *Griswold et al v Connecticut*, which dealt with an alleged infringement of the right of privacy in marriage. The Court established that, although privacy was not guaranteed in so many words by the Constitution or the Bill of Rights, it was a basic and fundamental right deeply rooted in our society. Justice Douglas delivered the opinion of the Court and discussed the idea that various other guarantees in the Constitution created zones of individual privacy.[87]

In the mid-1960s nurse investigators were just beginning to make inroads in biological research. Among other problems, the use of double-blind techniques—requiring the withholding of certain treatment information from both the patient and the staff caring for the patient— necessitates skilled handling to protect the subject. Such a situation requires value judgments grounded in professional ethics to determine the degree of risk compared with the potential benefits obtained. In the mid-1960s, the nature of consent to participate in research as a human subject could be implicit, explicit, or in the form of a written statement and, for example, the fact that a patient was admitted to a hospital implied a certain degree of implicit consent. With the advent of governmental guidelines for the use of human subjects and the establishment of peer review committees to assist in safeguarding the rights of human subjects through a formal informed consent procedure, the informal and blanket mechanisms, which could be too easily abused, became ancient history.

In 1969, Berthold wrote a detailed paper based on a review of the literature and focused on the larger topic of maintaining human rights and values amidst a scientific–technological revolution and the concomitant social revolution. She developed the idea that the right of the individual in American society to dignity, self-respect, and freedom of self-determination has been in conflict with the rights and long-range interests of society on many occasions and on various issues. Berthold went on to say that these conflicts have generally been characterized as involving humanitarian, libertarian, and scientific values. Humanitarian values have to do with respect for the sanctity of human life and the safeguards needed to protect the subject from physical or emotional harm. Libertarian values have to do with the individual's political, civil, and individual rights to self-respect, dignity, freedom of thought and action, and the safeguards needed to protect the individual from invasion of his privacy without his knowledge for the sake of knowledge. Scientific values concern the safeguards needed to protect the right to know anything that may be known or discovered about any part of the universe. In specific situations these different values lead to competing moral claims that must be balanced against one another within the process of moral reasoning.[88]

Scientific inquiry can involve several specific ethical issues, all of which should be considered by the nurse investigator when designing the research as well as by the potential human subject giving informed consent. These issues include: (1) loss of dignity and autonomy; (2) invasion of privacy; (3) time and energy requirements; (4) mental and physical discomfort or pain; and (5) risk of physical or emotional injury. These issues must be weighed against potential benefits for the subject himself, for people like him (e.g., diabetics), and for the general good of all people.

In 1970, Batey raised the question as to when and to what extent the issue of the rights of human subjects becomes a methodological issue in nursing research. She made the point that researchers have historically been accorded considerable prestige; however, fewer and fewer people now respond compliantly and with unquestioning deference to others who hold prestigious positions. She also asked whether there is a metaprofessional ethic or a set of values guiding nurse researchers—who are both researchers and clinicians. In addition, she asked whether nurse researchers share a set of values directed toward optimizing the conditions needed for fulfillment of the aims of science.[89]

The American Nurses' Association (ANA) has been active in developing guidelines on ethical values for the nurse in research. In 1968, the Committee on Research and Studies said that nursing was committed to the identification and elaboration of a body of scientific knowledge specific to nursing represented by the descriptive, explanatory, and predictive principles that guide nursing practice for the provision of optimal nursing services to society. The ANA reaffirmed its belief in the rights and the responsibilities of members of the profession to conduct research and to meet its obligations to those members by establishing guidelines on ethical values. In discussing these ethical dimensions within the framework of protecting human rights, the ANA elaborated on the rights to privacy, to self-determination, to conservation of personal resources, to freedom from arbitrary hurt, and to freedom from intrinsic risk of injury. The rights of minors and incompetent persons, such as young children or unconscious patients, and the informed consent process were also discussed. Essentially, the ANA's position rests on the idea that the relationship of trust between subject and investigator requires that the subject be assured that he will be treated fairly and that no discomfort, risk, or inconvenience, beyond that initially stated in obtaining informed consent, will be imposed without further permission being obtained from the subject.[90]

With this preliminary work on guidelines serving as a background, the ANA acknowledged the changes that had occurred in the early 1970s in the area of research regulations and guidelines for informed consent by publishing a position paper on human rights developed by the Commission on Nursing Research. One very important aspect of this document is its statement on human rights for the nurse.[91]

Implementation of this guideline implies the need for written statements about conditions of employment and any special expectations about work performance above and beyond that usually expected of a person occupying the position of nurse. In advance of such employment, nurses need to know if they will be expected to provide medicine, treatment, and other procedures as part of double-blind investigations. They need to know in advance if the work requires them to function as data collectors for research in addition to their role as nurses engaged in the delivery of patient care services. Conditions of employment must also provide for the option of not participating in clinical research if these work expectations are not spelled out in advance of employment.*

The nurse who conducts research does not differ from her colleagues in other disciplines. Her research protocol and activities must ensure that the human subject will be informed in understandable language and will in no way be coerced to participate or continue in the study but will be free to exercise his freedom of self-determination. As stated previously, the integrity and the ethics of the investigator will safeguard the safety and the rights of the human subject. The patient's safety and his rights must be attended to within the context of the advancement of nursing knowledge, the growing number of nurses engaged in an academic or a research career, and the rising professionalism of nursing. Nursing needs a fuller discussion within the profession of the issues involved in research with human subjects, informed consent, and the conflicting moral claims that create ethical dilemmas for the nurse researcher who is the principle investigator and for the nurse in the clinical setting who assists in another's research. The issue of informed consent was explored in detail in the first book on ethics and nursing research, *Patients, Nurses, Ethics*, by Davis and Krueger.[92]

The nurse's ethical obligation in informed consent and treatment protocols for patients is to ascertain whether the patient understands what he has been told and what he has been consented to. Since informed consent is an imperfect tool, patients may have questions about their treatment that indicate that they do not fully understand what is going on.[93] Even if the patients do not initiate this subject, the nurse needs to find out if they actually do understand the nature of the treatment regimen.

Several articles have addressed informed consent and nursing.[94-102] Data-based papers on the role of nurses in the informed consent process reveal some interesting findings.[103-105] For example, one of these studies identified five roles in which nurses have assumed active involvement in informed consent. These roles are: (1) watchdog to monitor informed consent situations; (2) advocate to mediate on behalf of patients; (3) resource person to provide information on alternatives; (4) coordinator to preserve an open, friendly atmosphere for discussion; and (5) facilitator to clarify differences between involved parties. Such studies raise the larger issue of disclosure of information in informed consent. Questions arise about how much information should be disclosed, what information, and who disclosed it. One study on the attitudes of nurses and medical students toward nurses disclosing

---

Reprinted with permission of the American Nurses' Association.

information to patients pointed to areas of possible conflict. Generally, this conflict can be seen as one between a strong view of patients' rights and the need of hospital bureaucracies to maintain orderly channels of communication.[106]

Once the nurse has discovered that the patient does not understand aspects of the treatment, her ethical obligation is to report this to the physician so that he can meet his ethical obligations to inform. Usually physicians follow through and speak further with patients regarding their treatment. If a physician decides not to provide additional information, however, or not to clarify what has already been said, the question arises as to the nurse's obligation in the situation. Has the nurse met her professional obligation when she tells the physician that the patient needs additional input about his treatment, or does she need to do something more when the physician does not follow through? The basic question here has to do with the extent of the nurse's obligation in matters of informed consent.

In situations where information is withheld from patients, the nurse must ethically reason through to some conclusion, and on that basis she will decide the ethical thing to do. It is important to remember that ethical dilemmas may not have been solved merely by replacing the physician's values with the nurse's. The central question is what does the patient want, or if the patient cannot make his position known because of his physical or mental status, then, who is to speak in his best interest?

REFERENCES

1. Kant I: *Groundwork of the Metaphysics of Morals.* New York: Harper Torchbooks; 1964.
2. Capron A: Informed consent in catastrophic disease and treatment. *University of Pennsylvania Law Rev* 123:364–376, December 1974.
3. Beauchamp TL, Childress JF: *Principles of Biomedical Ethics.* 2nd ed. New York; Oxford University Press, 1983.
4. Norton BG: *The Preservation of Species: The Value of Biological Diversity.* Princeton, NJ: Princeton University Press; 1986.
5. Donnelley S: Speculative philosophy, the troubled middle, and the ethics of animal experimentation. *Hastings Cent Rep* 19:15–21, March–April 1989.
6. Bernard C: *An Introduction to the Study of Experimental Medicine.* New York: Macmillan; 1927.
7. *Fortner v Koch.* 272 Mich 273, 282, 261, NW (Mich 1935).
8. Faden RR, Beauchamp, J: *A History and Theory of Informed Consent.* New York: Oxford University Press; 1986.
9. *Grants Administration Manual.* U.S. Department of Health, Education and Welfare; 1971.
10. Langer E: Human experimentation: New York verdict affirms patients' rights. *Science* 159:663–666, February 1966.

11. Krugman S, Giles JP: Viral hepatitis: New light on an old disease. *JAMA* 215:1019–1021, May 11 1970.
12. *Final Report of the Tuskegee Syphilis Study Ad Hoc Advisory Panel.* US Public Health Service; 1973.
13. President's Commission: *Making Health Care Decisions.* US Government Printing Office; October 1982.
14. Beecher HK: Ethics and clinical research. *N Engl J Med* 274:1354–1360, June 16, 1966.
15. Barber B: The ethics of experimentation with human subjects. *Sci Am* 234:25–31, February 1976.
16. Gray BH: *Human Subjects in Medical Experimentation.* New York: Wiley; 1975.
17. Jonas H: Philosophical reflections on experimenting with human subjects. In Freund PA (ed): *Experimentation with Human Subjects.* New York: Braziller; 1969: pp 1–31.
18. Parsons T: *The Social System.* Glencoe, IL: Free Press; 1951: p 437.
19. Alfidi RJ: Informed consent: A study of patient reaction. *JAMA* 216:1325–1329, May 24, 1971.
20. Baumrind D: Principles of ethical conduct in the treatment of subjects. *Am Psychol* 27:1083, November 1973.
21. Milgram S: Some conditions of obedience and disobedience to authority. *Hum Relations* 18:57–75, February 1965.
22. Hofling C, Brotzman E, Dalrymple S, et al: An experimental study in nurse–patient relationships. *J Nerv Ment Dis* 143:171–180, 1966.
23. Humphreys L: *Tearoom Trade: Impersonal Sex in Public Places.* Chicago: Aldine; 1970.
24. Rosenhan DL: On being sane in insane places. *Science* 167:250–258, January 19, 1973.
25. Lurie A: *Imaginary Friends*, New York: Avon; 1975.
26. Applebaum PS: *Informed Consent: Legal Theory and Clinical Practice.* New York: Oxford University Press; 1987.
27. Cross AN, Churchill LR: Ethical and cultural dimensions of informed consent. *Ann Intern Med* 96:110–113, January 1982.
28. Lidz CW, Meisel JD, Osterweis M et al: Barriers to informed consent. *Ann Intern Med* 99:539–543, October 1983.
29. Grim PS, Singer PA, Gramelspacher GP et al.: Informed consent in emergency research. *JAMA* 262:252–255, July 14, 1989.
30. Svensson CK: Representation of American Blacks in clinical trials of new drugs. *JAMA* 261:263–265. January 13, 1989.
31. Baker MT, Taub HA: Readability of informed consent forms for research in a veterans administration medical center. *JAMA* 250:2646–2648, November 18, 1983.
32. Riecken HW, Ravick R: Informed consent to biomedical research in veterans administration hospitals. *JAMA* 248:344–348, July 16, 1982.
33. Appelbaum PS, Grisso T: Assessing patients' capacities to consent to treatment. *N Engl J Med* 319:1635–1638, December 22, 1988.
34. Capron AM: Medical research in prisons. *Hastings Cent Rep* 3:4–6, June 1973.
35. Mitford J: Experimentation behind bars. *Atlantic Monthly* January 1973, pp 64–73.

36. Jonsen A, Parker M, Carlson R, Emmett C: *Biomedical Experimentation on Prisoners: Review of Practices and Problems and Proposal of a New Regulatory Approach.* San Francisco: University of California, School of Medicine, Health Policy Program; September 1975.
37. Burt RA: Why we should keep prisoners from the doctors: Reflections on the Detroit psychosurgery case. *Hastings Cent Rep* 5:25–34, February 1975.
38. Mitchell A: Research with women prisoners. In Davis AJ, Krueger JC (eds): *Patients, Nurses, Ethics.* New York: Am J Nurs Co, 1980: pp 129–135.
39. Dyer AR, Block S: Informed consent and the psychiatric patients. *J Med Ethics* 13:12–16, 1989.
40. Pothier PC: Ethics and research on children. In Davis AJ, Krueger JC (eds): *Patients, Nurses, Ethics* New York: Am J Nurs Co, 1980: pp 149–162.
41. McCormick RA: Proxy consent in the experimentation situation. *Persp in Biol and Med* Autumn 1974, pp 2–20.
42. Lowe CU, Alexander D, Mishkin B, et al.: Nontherapeutic research on children: An ethical dilemma. *J Pediatr* 84:468–473, April 1974.
43. Fowler MDM: Pediatric informed consent. *Heart Lung,* 17:584–585, September 1988.
44. Sorenson JH, Bergman GE: Delineating paternalism in pediatric care. *Theor Med* 5:93–104, May 1984.
45. Kass L: Babies by means of vitro fertilization: Unethical experiments on the unborn? *N Engl J Med* pp 1174–1178, November 18, 1971.
46. Reback GL: Fetal experimentation: Moral, legal, and medical implications. *Stanford Law Rev* pp 1191–1207, May 1974.
47. Fost N: Our curious attitudes toward the fetus. *Hastings Cent Rep* 4:4–5, February 1974.
48. Dykes MHM, Czapek EE: Regulations and legislation concerning abortus research. *JAMA* 219:1303–1304, September 2, 1974.
49. Curran WJ: Experimentation becomes a crime: Fetal research in Massachusetts. *N Engl J Med* 293:300–301, February 6, 1975.
50. Caylin W. Lappé M: Fetal politics: The debate on experimenting with the unborn. *Atlantic Monthly* 95:66–73, May 1975.
51. Hart DS: Fetal research and antiabortion politics: Holding science hostage. *Fam Plann Perspect* 4:72–82, March–April 1975.
52. Lappé M: The moral claims of the wanted fetus. *Hastings Cent Rep* 5: 11–14, April 1975.
53. Powledge TM: Fetal experimentation: Sorting out the issues. *Hastings Cent Rep* 5:8–10, April 1975.
54. Ramsey P: *The Ethics of Fetal Research.* New Haven: Yale University Press; 1975.
55. Fost N, Chudwin D, Wikler D: The limited moral significance of fetal viability. *Hastings Cent Rep* 10:10–13, December 1980.
56. Grobstein C: *Science and the Unborn.* New York: Basic Books; 1988.
57. Culliton B: White House wants fetal research ban. *Science* 217:1423, September 16, 1988.
58. Fletcher J, Ryan K: Federal regulations for fetal research: A case for reform. *Law, Med Health Care* 15:126–128, Fall 1987.
59. Butler RN: *Why Survive? Being Old in America.* New York: Harper & Row; 1975.

60. Ratzan RM: Being old makes you different: The ethics of research with elderly subjects. *Hastings Cent Rep* 10:32–42, October 1980.
61. Stanley B, Guido MA, Stanley M, Shortell D: The elderly patient and informed consent. *JAMA* 252:1302–1306, September 14, 1984.
62. Marston RQ: Research on minors, prisoners and the mentally ill. *N Engl J Med* 291:158–159, January 18, 1973.
63. Childress JF: Compensating injured research subjects: The moral arguments. *Hastings Cent Rep* 6:21–27, December 1976.
64. Lund CC: The doctor, the patient and the truth. *Ann Intern Med* 24:955–959, March 1978.
65. Cabot RC: The use of truth and falsehood in medicine. *Conn Med* 42:189–194, March 1978.
66. Becker AH, Weisman AD: The patient with a fatal illness: To tell or not to tell. *JAMA*, 212:152–154, August 21, 1967.
67. Fletcher J: *Morals and Medicine.* Princeton, NJ: Princeton University Press; 1954: pp 34–64.
68. Besch L: Informed consert: A patient's right. *Nurs Outlook* 31:32–35, January 1979.
69. Meyer BC: Truth and the physician. *Bull NY Acad Med* 45:59–71, January 1969.
70. Kelly LY: The patient's right to know. *Nurs Outlook* 26:26–32, January 1976.
71. Hanganu E, Popa G: Cancer and truth. *J Med Ethics* 3:74–75, 1977.
72. Minogue BP, Taraszewski R: The whole truth and nothing but the truth? *Hastings Cent Rep* 18:34–36, October–November 1988.
73. Kelly WD, Friesen SR: Do cancer patients want to be told? *Surgery* 27:822–826, June 1950.
74. Bowen OR: Why cancer victims should be told the truth. *Med Times* 83:793–799, August 1955.
75. Samp RJ, Curreri AR: A questionnaire survey on public cancer education obtained from cancer patients and their families. *Cancer* 10:382–384, . March–April 1957.
76. Dodge JS: How much should the patient be told—and by whom? *Hospitals* 37:66–79, 125, December 16, 1963.
77. Linehan DT: What does the patient want to know? *Am J Nurs* 66:1066–1070, May 1966.
78. Alfidi RJ: Informed consent: A study of patient reaction. *JAMA* 216:1325–1329, May 24, 1971.
79. Dodge JS: What patients should be told. *Am J Nurs* 72:1852–1854, October 1972.
80. Marsh FH: An ethical approach to paternalism in the physician–patient relationship. *Ethics Sci Med* 4:135–138, 1977.
81. Kant I: *Groundwork of the Metaphysics of Morals.*
82. Downie RS, Telfer E: Respect for persons. New York: Schocken Books; 1970: pp 14–15.
83. Carpenter WT: The nurse's role in informed consent. *Nurs Times* 71:1049–1051, July 3, 1975.
84. Hubbard S, DeVita V: Chemotherapy research: The nurse in oncology. *Am J Nurs* 76:560–565, April 1976.
85. Jacobson SF: Ethical issues in experimentation with human subjects. *Nurs Forum* 12(1):58–71, 1973.

86. Abdellah FG: Approaches to protecting the rights of human subjects. *Nurs Res*, Fall 1967, pp 316–320.
87. *Griswold et al v Connecticut*, 381 US 479 (1965).
88. Berthold JS: Advancement of science and technology while maintaining human rights and values. *Nurs Res*, 18:514–522, November–December 1969.
89. Batey MV: Some methodological issues in research. *Nurs Res* 19:511–516, November–December 1970.
90. ANA Committee on Research and Studies: The nurse in research: ANA guidelines on ethical values. *Nurs Res* 17:104–107, March–April 1968.
91. ANA Commission on Nursing Research: *Human Rights Guidelines for Nurses in Clinical and Other Research*. Kansas City, MO: American Nurses' Association; 1975.
92. Davis AJ, Krueger JC: *Patients, Nurses, Ethics*. New York: American Journal of Nursing Co.; 1980.
93. Cassileth B, Zupkis R, Sutton-Smith K, et al: Informed consent: Why are its goals imperfectly realized? *N Engl J Med* 298:896–899, April 17, 1980.
94. Weikel C: Informed consent: An ethical dilemma–the nurse's role. *Today's OR Nurse* 5:10, January 1987.
95. Walker, CL: Informed consent with children. *J Assoc Pediatr Oncol Nurses* 5:38–40, May 1988.
96. Brooke PS: Informed consent: An ethical dilemma having life/death and legal implications. *Clin Nurse Specialist* 2:157–161, Fall 1988.
97. Schoen DC: Ethical issues in nursing research. *Orthop Nurs* 3:47, July–August 1988.
98. Woods SL: Informed consent in research and the critically ill adult. *Prog Cardiovasc Nurs* 9:89–92, July–September 1988.
99. White BC: Ethical issues surrounding informed consent: A brief history and ethical foundations surrounding informed consent. *Urol Nurs* 9:11–14, January–March 1989.
100. White BC: Ethical issues surrounding informed consent: Components of a morally valid consent and conditions that impair its validity. *Urol Nurs* 9:4–9, April–June 1989.
101. Case NK: Substitutive judgment in the pediatric health care setting. *Issues Compr Pediatr Nurs* 11:303–312, September–October 1988.
102. Davis AJ, Underwood PR: The competency quagmire: Clarification of the nursing perspective concerning the issue of competence and informed consent. *Int J Nurs Stud* 26:271–279, 1989.
103. Davis AJ: The clinical nurse's role in informed consent. *J Prof Nurs* 4:88–91, March/April 1988.
104. Davis AJ: Informed consent process in research protocols: Dilemmas for clinical nurses. *West J Nurs Res* 11:448–457, August 1989.
105. Davis AJ: Clinical nurses ethical decision making in situations of informed consent. *Adv Nurs* 11:63–69, April 1989.
106. Davis AJ, Jameton A: Nursing and medical student attitudes toward nursing disclosure of information to patients: A pilot study. *J Adv Nurs* 12:691–698, December 1987.

CHAPTER **8**

Abortion

ETHICS AND REPRODUCTIVE TECHNOLOGY

The field of reproductive technology has exploded over the past few years. Neonatal intensive care is a dramatic example of high-technology medicine and nursing. Embryo freezing as an adjunct to in vitro fertilization (IVF) is a large step forward in the treatment of infertility and control of human reproduction. Technologies such as artificial insemination, IVF, surrogate motherhood, and ovum transfer raise numerous ethical issues. Fetal research as one part of these developments has received much attention as an ethical concern in public policy. The experimental drug, RU 486, used to terminate early pregnancy, raises again the question about the status of the early embryo. And yet, with all these scientific developments and the attending ethical dilemmas raised by them, it is the ancient act of abortion that holds center stage in the debates.

ABORTION AND BIRTH CONTROL

The battle over abortion, sometimes called the battle of life versus choice, has become one of the most emotional issues of politics and morality facing the United States today. The language used in this debate is so passionate and polemical, and the conflicting and seemingly irreconcilable values so deeply felt, that this issue could well test the very foundations of a pluralistic system of government that was designed to accommodate deep-rooted moral and ethical differences. It is possible that nothing since the issue of slavery has the potential of dividing us in our quest for a democratic society as does abortion. Some believe that abortion is murder of the unborn person and therefore should be outlawed by constitutional amendment. Others argue that abortion is a right that women must have legally because they must be free to control their bodies and their lives. Along with the ethical dilemma of abortion itself, another issue, that of the government's role, has become paramount. Should abortion be legal or illegal? If legal, should government funds be available to cover the cost of abortion for the poor? The abortion issue promises to be the political battle of the 1990s.

Since the 1973 Supreme Court decision on abortion, the annual number of abortions performed in this country has increased from 744,600 to 1,500,000.

Abortion has become a topic of great national debate at all levels of government and in other arenas, both religious and secular. There has been an organized attempt to overturn the 1973 Supreme Court decision to legalize abortion. Few other recent topics have caused so much outcry and activity, although antinuclear sentiments may do so in the near future. One side of the debate has been called The Right to Life, while the other side has come to be known as The Right to Choice. Many people take a position somewhere between these two stances but are not so visible or vocal in their stance. The ethical dilemmas in abortion are complex and require that we examine them carefully. It seems reasonable to assume that such an examination will need to take into account the social and religious diversity in the United States and to recall that a major philosophical basis here is the separation of church and state.

The 1973 *Roe v Wade* decision by the majority of seven to two of the Supreme Court justices asserted that the constitutional right to privacy is broad enough to encompass a woman's decision whether or not to terminate her pregnancy. The right to abortion was determined to be fundamental; therefore the state could intervene only if it could demonstrate a compelling state interest. Two compelling state interests were stated by the Court: (1) protection of maternal health; and (2) the potential of human life, but only as the pregnancy progressed. Regulations to protect the health of the mother are compelling only when there is more danger for the woman to have an abortion than to carry the fetus to term. Protecting fetal life is compelling only when the fetus is viable.

Efforts to overturn the 1973 *Roe v Wade* decision by constitutional amendments have failed, but another strategy, the passage of state abortion statutes that are as restrictive as possible according to the *Roe v Wade* framework, aims to see the Supreme Court ultimately modify or abandon *Roe* altogether. In January 1989, the Court heard a case involving a Missouri statute designed to restrict access to abortion. The position of the Missouri legislature included: (1) the life of each human being begins at conception; (2) hospitalization is required for abortions; (3) a physician is required to determine viability in a pregnancy of 20 weeks or more by performing specific tests; (4) there is to be no use of public funds, which included prohibiting counseling women to have abortions and not allowing physicians to perform privately paid abortions in public facilities. The Supreme Court did not uphold every aspect of this position. Important for our consideration is the question of what the Missouri case, known as *Reproductive Health Services v Webster* (1988), means in the larger sense. One legal scholar says that all these disputes are about whether women (and their physicians) or state legislatures make decisions regarding abortions. For the court to permit states to outlaw abortion, the most frequently performed medical procedure in the United States, seems unlikely but a narrowing of *Roe* seems inevitable. This narrowing will likely add restrictions to minors seeking abortions and confine abortions to earlier points in pregnancy.[1]

Abortion, the expulsion or removal of the products of conception from the uterus, generally occurs before the 28th week of pregnancy. Spontaneous abortion occurs as a result of a variety of endogenous and exogenous causes, excluding intentional human interference. Such human interference, called induced abortion, to deliberately terminate a pregnancy, performed either legally or illegally, relies on a number of different methods. The method used depends, in part, on timing, or how long the pregnancy has existed. Medically speaking, abortion during the first trimester is easiest to perform and safest for the woman involved. However, women do undergo abortion during the second trimester or until the fetus becomes viable. Viability of the fetus means that it has potential ability to live outside the uterus, albeit with artificial means, if necessary. Traditionally, viability was thought to occur around 28 weeks, but developments in technology have begun to move the time to an earlier date in the pregnancy. In the last trimester, abortion presents increased dangers to the woman, and the likelihood of delivering a live fetus also increases.

Statistically speaking, abortion—one of the world's oldest and most popular methods of birth control, if performed under good conditions early in pregnancy—has become safer than carrying a baby to full term. Critics have challenged previous comparisons of mortality from legal abortions and childbirth, saying they contrast population groups with different clinical characteristics. To address this issue, a research team calculated standardized abortion and childbirth mortality rates between 1972 and 1978 while adjusting for preexisting medical conditions to make the two groups comparable. The findings indicated that between 1972 and 1978, woman were about seven times more likely to die from childbirth than from legal abortion.[2] Another research team reviewed the sources of mortality data on which these comparisons are based and examined the completeness and accuracy of both sets of statistics. They concluded that the crude data are biased in a direction that overestimates the abortion risks for the women relative to the risks of childbearing.[3] The argument can be made that other effective methods of contraception have been developed that could replace abortion as a means of birth control in most cases. Furthermore, these alternatives to abortion have the potential of presenting fewer ethical dilemmas for many who use them. Several factors must be taken into account before pursuing this line of argument very far, however. First, not all people receive sound knowledge about sex and reproduction, and in many places people still continue to do battle over sex education in the schools. Second, research findings have begun to throw into question the safety of the most effective birth control device, the pill. And finally, the fact remains that people do not necessarily act on information and knowledge they have, even when the results of their actions may prove detrimental to their health or lives. For example, behaviors such as smoking, driving while intoxicated, and having sexual intercourse without using some form of contraception when the couple does not want a pregnancy all support this fact. Contraceptive devices succeed in preventing unwanted pregnancies only if used consistently. The nature of human sexuality and the complex motivations that people bring to their sexual experiences favor mishaps. For these and other reasons not discussed here, abortion as a form of birth control remains with us.

BACKGROUND

Inevitably, the statistical data on legal or illegal abortions performed in the past cannot be stated with certainty. One study of legal abortion covering the years 1957 through 1962, when there were far more restrictions than after 1973, indicated that the women questioned had 1039 abortions as against 522,600 live births. This means there existed a ratio of about two abortions to every 1000 live births. Using this ratio and extrapolating it to about 4,000,000 deliveries yearly in this country, we could make an educated guess, that, for the years of the study, approximately 8000 legal abortions were performed annually.[4] We have, for obvious reasons, even fewer facts about illegal abortions. However, some observations have been made that suggest certain patterns and concerns. In the United States before the 1973 Supreme Court decision, abortion was largely performed clandestinely by physicians, especially for the financially well off. The poor were more likely to abort, themselves, or to resort to nonmedical amateurs. As well as we can determine, the majority of those fetuses aborted were from married women with several children. Death and invalidism have not been inconsiderable as an aftermath of illegal abortion. In the 1960s, almost 50 percent of deaths in New York City associated with pregnancy and birth resulted form illegal abortions.[5] The death rate from abortion in Hungary, where women can easily obtain a legal abortion, has been reported as less than 6 per 100,000. In the United States, the death rate resulting from the removal of tonsils and adenoids has been put at 17 per 100,000, while the death rate from childbirth and its complications has been reported as 24 per 100,000.[6] The past 35 years have seen a downward trend in both reported maternal mortality, excluding abortion, and reported mortality from abortion. These declines primarily reflect progress in the prevention and treatment of puerperal infection and other complications associated with pregnancy and childbirth. In these years of declining mortality rates, mortality from abortion in the United States remained much higher among nonwhite women than among white women.[7]

Numerous regional and national studies conducted during the last 20 years indicate that the poor, the less educated, and blacks want about the same number of children as others in this society.[8-12] Despite the desire for relatively small families, the studies also show that these groups tend to have larger families than they want. At every point of choice, the middle- and upper-class white woman has tended to have greater access to contraception, abortion, forced marriage, and adoption. Prior to the 1973 abortion law, research data collected in those states where repeal laws had been passed demonstrated that when abortion became more readily available, the lower socioeconomic groups made the greatest use of abortion facilities.[13-15]

One of the reasons given in the past for not making abortions accessible has been the psychiatric concern that such a traumatic procedure would lead to a burden of guilt and possibly to mental illness. Such statements rarely could be supported by reliable scientific evidence involving a large sample. One psychiatrist, as early as 1970, found in a careful review of the literature that little justification for this traditional opinion existed. Another psychiatrist referred to the myth of serious emotional sequelae but went on to say that even psychiatric illness is no reason to deny a woman an abortion. In his experience, most normal women respond to abortion with mild feelings of depression while mentally ill women respond with improved mental attitudes. More recently, in 1989, a report from the Surgeon General's office indicated that data were lacking to support the notion that abortions were harmful to women who had them. This report received attention in newspapers and on radio and television around the country. Both the social and psychological dimensions of abortion require further study. These dimensions interact with the general attitudes toward abortion held by society, including those of health professionals.

Although change seems inevitable and rapid, attitudes do take time to shift on many important issues. Approximately seven national surveys conducted between 1962 and 1969 on attitudes toward abortion showed that public opinion changed very little during these eight years. Although the abortion controversy came into sharp focus during the 1960s and the underlying issues had been with us for many years, not until 1972 did a survey show more favorable public attitudes toward abortion.[19] Public opinion on abortion has in a general sense been fairly stable since the 1973 decision, with the majority supporting the decision.[20] However, it is important to understand that the public does not necessarily approve of abortion under all circumstances, as is the case with *Roe v Wade*. In January 1985, *Newsweek* published a poll in which 21 percent of the respondents stated that they believed abortion should be legal under all circumstances, 22 percent illegal under all circumstances, while 54 percent believed that it should be legal under only certain circumstances. Although some physicians have favored the liberalized abortion laws, others oppose them. Reluctance, if not downright opposition, has characterized the attitude of some physicians. The influence of this segment of the medical profession on whether women find abortions more difficult or easier to obtain becomes a critical factor. Data indicate that in 1976 approximately 700,000 women wanted abortions but were unable to obtain them. Furthermore, only 27 percent of all general non-Catholic hospitals in the country performed abortions.[21] Recent attempts to change the abortion law may impact this situation further.

The development of a number of other medical procedures is having an influence on abortion as a birth control measure. Not without their own ethical and legal issues, sterilization and artificial insemination have received more publicity in recent years and may develop into practical alternatives for controlling pregnancy. Amniocentesis, the procedure whereby a sample of amniotic fluid can be obtained for analysis, may eventually become a routine part of good prenatal care. In the mid-1960s, there began an almost imperceptible shift in the focus of amniocentesis from a tool used in the latter stages of pregnancy to detect and treat abnormalities to a means of early detection and abortion. This change has been received with positive reactions by those who view the procedure as a means of treating abnormalities in utero, or who see opportunities for early detection and abortion of an abnormal fetus when treatment cannot be undertaken. Others, however, have raised the question of the myriad of ethical dilemmas that surround the procedure. One writer puts it succinctly when he says that the lure of a genetic test for a normal—and possibly in the future, an optimal—infant threatens to reinforce a trend in our society toward eugenics, relegating the less-than-optimal fetuses into categories for assortment and ultimate disposal.[22] Other technologies will allow the detection of a normal fetus even earlier than can now be obtained with amniocentesis. These clinical tools are being developed and marketed.

A great many factors intersect in any discussion of abortion: medical, sociological, psychological, technological, and the attitudes grounded in philosophical and moral concerns that the public has developed. This background information, along with the overview of the historical and social context of abortion to follow, will help us to understand more fully the ethical dilemmas surrounding abortion.

THE LARGER CONTEXT

According to the decree of the United States Supreme Court in 1973, abortion is a lawful act during the first trimester of pregnancy. After the first trimester, the state can restrict abortion through regulations protecting the pregnant woman's health. The state may regulate or forbid abortion after viability except in those instances where medical judgments indicate its necessity to safeguard the health or life of the pregnant woman. The lawyer arguing *Roe v Wade* before the Court traced the legal history of abortion. The restrictive criminal abortion laws in effect at the time the Court heard the case derived from statutory changes mainly effected during the latter half of the 19th century. A brief historical view of religious attitudes, the law, and scientific and social developments form the larger context within which to understand the Court's decision regarding abortion.

Historical Context

At the time of the Persian Empire, abortifacients were accessible, though individuals who performed criminal abortions received severe punishment. In ancient Greece and during the Roman era, people resorted to abortion without scruple.[23] Plato in *The Republic* and Aristotle in *Politics* described abortion as a means of preventing excess population. Neither Greek nor Roman law afforded protection to the unborn fetus. Furthermore, the religions practiced in these cultures did not bar abortion; however, philosophers, religious teachers, and physicians debated the morality of performing abortions. In this climate, the Hippocratic Oath developed and took a position against abortion. One theory explains this radical departure from the prevailing practice of the time in light of Pythagorean dogma.[24] Most Greek thinkers, except for the Pythagorean school, commended abortion, at least prior to viability. For the Pythagoreans, the embryo became animated or infused with a soul from the moment of conception, so that abortion meant destroying a living being. The abortion clause in the Hippocratic Oath reflects Pythagorean doctrine, a small segment of Greek opinion at the time. Furthermore, medical writings down to Galen's time (AD 130–200) provided evidence of violation of almost every injunction of the oath. For example, Soranos (AD 98–138), a Greek from Ephesus, became Rome's leading gynecologist, and in his writings he lists the reasons for abortion and the means to achieve it.[25] Only at the end of antiquity, with the emerging teachings of Christianity, which agreed with the Pythagorean ethic, did the oath become the nucleus of all medical ethics and become regarded as the embodiment of truth. For some, this historical context explains what appears to them as the rigidity of the Hippocratic Oath.

The Greco-Roman world, distinguished by its indifference to fetal life, also saw the development of Christianity, which gave rise to values in opposition to and conflict with the generally held popular beliefs. The specific Christian teaching on abortion developed within a theological context of the Christian valuation of life, grounded in the Old Testament command to love your neighbor as yourself (Levitticus 19:18). The basis for fulfillment of this commandment, found in the New Testament, emphasized the sacrifice of a man's life for another (John 15:13). From this commandment of love, the Christian valuation of life evolved.[26]

Abortion, as a subject of concern to secular humanists and theologians, has a long history. At the heart of this complex discourse lies the question of how one determines the humanity of a being. The Roman Catholic position on abortion has been clearly stated since the late 1880s and has been reaffirmed by recent popes. Roman Catholics, as well as some other religious leaders, believe the embryo becomes a human being with a soul from the moment of conception. Some of the early teachers of the Church, however, including St. Thomas Aquinas, did not consider it possible for an unformed embryo to have a soul and placed ensoulment at about three months after conception, when the fetus had developed a recognizable human shape. Along with this concept of ensoulment at conception, Roman Catholics reject abortion on the grounds that unborn children need baptism. Although not as strongly upheld in the Church today, this doctrine of baptizing the endangered fetus still holds. The current official position of Catholic leaders accepts the concept of ensoulment that defines the fetus as a human being from conception. This position can be characterized as a refusal to discriminate among human beings on the basis of their varying potentialities.

Protestant views vary according to the numerous sects and groups involved. Although many Protestants do not agree with the Roman Catholic Church on ensoulment, they do regard abortion as undesirable, though not a mortal sin, since the embryo as an entity should be preserved from unnecessary destruction. Generally, for Protestants, the concept of the sacredness of life has served as an obstacle to the wanton and thoughtless performance of abortion. In attempting to determine when human life begins, most Protestant leaders agree that by the time of quickening, or the first recognizable movements of the fetus in utero, one can define the fetus as a human being.

One Protestant writer outlined pertinent principles that can be stipulated for reflection and reduced them to the following simplified scheme. First, life must be preserved rather than destroyed; second, protection must be provided, especially to those who cannot assert their own right to life; and third, exceptions to these rules exist, such as (1) medical indications that make therapeutic abortion morally tolerable; (2) pregnancy resulting from a sexual crime; (3) social and emotional conditions that do not appear beneficial for the well-being of the mother and child.[27] This writer replaced the determination of an action as right or wrong according to its conformity to a rule and its application with stressing the primacy of the person and human relationships along with the concreteness of the choice within limited possibilities. In the case of abortion, he maintained that no guarantee of an objectively right action can be given, since several values, all objectively important, exist. Furthermore, these values do not resolve themselves into a harmonious relationship to each other. Since there is no single overriding determination of what constitutes a right action, there can be no unambiguously right act.[28]

Ancient Jewish writings consider the fetus a living being when it detaches itself from the mother. According to the Talmud, this occurs when the head has emerged from the birth canal. In more modern times, Orthodox Jewish leaders maintain that abortion is morally wrong at any time, except when the mother's life becomes seriously threatened. Reform Jews accept more reasons for abortion. For all practical purposes, the relatively permissive attitudes of Conservative and Reform Judaism can be equated with those of a growing number of Protestant sects on the topic of abortion.[29]

To briefly summarize the attitudes of the other great religions, Buddhists condemn killing but define commencement of life rather loosely, whereas the Shinto religion recognizes the infant as a living being after birth. The Islamic religion takes the stance that abortion is permissible until the embryo develops into the human shape, or for 120 days after conception.[30]

Legal Context

The legal aspects of abortion have been influenced by religious developments and definitions. In the fourth century AD, the Roman Empire developed the first laws against abortion in a time when Christian influence began to be felt. However, in the common law, abortion performed prior to quickening, at 16 to 18 weeks, was not an indictable offense.[31] This lack of criminality in common law for abortion occurring before quickening seems to have been influenced by theological concepts, civil and canonical law concepts, and philosophical concepts of the beginning of life, of when the embryo becomes infused with a soul. Christian theology and canon law fixed the point of animation at 40 days for a male and 80 days for a female, a view that persisted until the 19th century. General agreement developed that prior to animation, the fetus was part of the mother and therefore its destruction was not homicide. However, because of the uncertainty as to the exact time of animation and perhaps, influenced by Aquinas' definition of movement in utero as one criterion of life, Bracton wrote in 1640, in the first references to abortion in English criminal law, that to abort a woman is homicide if the embryo is formed and especially if it is animated.[32] Other English legal scholars, such as Edward Coke, Matthew Hale, and William Russell, used the concept of quickening to develop the common-law precedents regarding abortion. In 1803, England's first criminal abortion statute made the abortion of a quick fetus a capital crime. This law also provided lesser penalties for the felony of abortion that occurred before quickening. In 1967, the British Parliament enacted a new, liberal abortion law.

In the United States, generally speaking, the law in effect until the middle of the 19th century was the pre-existing English common law. These final statutes were lenient with abortion before quickening but dealt severely with abortion after quickening. During the middle and late 19th century, the quickening distinction disappeared from the statutory law in most states and the penalties for performing an abortion increased.[33] For approximately 100 years, the United States outlawed virtually all abortions. Some states made slight changes in their abortion laws before 1959; however, the movement toward definite reform, pioneered by Colorado, and based on the American Law Institute's Model Penal Code, occurred in 1967. Rather than creating an abortion-mill situation, as feared by its critics, this statute resulted in caution on the part of physicians and hospitals.[34]

The United States Supreme Court decision, delivered on January 22, 1973, declared both an original statute (Texas, *Roe v Wade*) and a reform statute (Georgia, *Doe v Bolton*) unconstitutional, ruling that a state could not interfere in the abortion decision between a woman and her physician during the first trimester. In the second trimester, when abortion becomes more hazardous, the state's interest in the woman's health permits the enactment of regulation to protect maternal health. Beyond these procedural requirements, the abortion decision still rests with the woman and her physician. After the fetus reaches viability, approximately in the last trimester, the state can exercise its interest in promoting potential human life. At this stage, the state can prohibit abortion except when the necessity arises to preserve the life or health of the mother. The Court did not support the position that a woman has an absolute right to abortion regardless of circumstances; however, the position it did take made legal abortion potentially more available than at any time in the United States during the 20th century. In 1976, the Court dealt with several additional issues regarding abortion, the consent of the spouse, the right of a minor to an abortion, and whether the state can stop a particular method of abortion.

The major grounds in the Court's decision evolved from the 14th Amendment of the Constitution and its concept of personal liberty and developed into the woman's right to privacy that, according to the Court, "is broad enough to encompass a woman's decision whether or not to terminate her pregnancy." As late as 1977, the proabortionists continued to fight to remove the remaining restriction in the abortion law, while the antiabortionists strove for a Constitutional amendment that would recognize a fetus's right to life. In light of its long history and the great passions generated by the abortion issue, continuation of this controversy can be expected in and out of legislatures and courts. The abortion laws prior to 1973 express a responsibility ethic that has been an important aspect of the psychosocial structure in this society. In effect, the laws have said that people are and must be responsible for the consequences of their acts; whether or not they are, they ought to be.[35]

Along with an ethic of responsibility, there has been much more recent debate on fetal rights from both a moral and a legal perspective. In fact, one writer maintains that there is a clear trend to expand fetal rights at the expense of pregnant women. This statement is backed up with the citation of numerous legal cases and the point is made that the legal system has begun to treat the maternal–fetal relationship as it does conflicts between two distinct and independent entities. That is, the law weighs the claims and interests of one against those of the other and then declares a winner. Such laws ignore the fact that the woman cannot walk away from the fetus and thereby avoid any restrictions or liabilities that the law might impose. In this created conflict, the state or another third party acts as the representative of the fetus.[36]

Medical Profession Context

The medical profession shared the antiabortion mood prevalent in the United States during the latter part of the 19th century and may have influenced the enactment of stringent criminal abortion legislation. In 1857 the American Medical Association (AMA) appointed a Committee on Criminal Abortion to investigate criminal abortion with a view to its general suppression. In 1859 this committee proposed, and the AMA adopted, a resolution against unwarrantable destruction of human life. They called upon state legislatures to revise their abortion laws and requested the cooperation of state medical societies in pressing the subject. The committee in 1871 again proposed resolutions that the AMA adopted. This time one recommendation read that it "be unlawful and unprofessional for any physician to induce abortion or premature labor without the concurrent opinion of at least one respectable consulting physician, and then always with a view to the safety of the child—if that be possible." They also recommended calling "the attention of the clergy of all denominations to the perverted views of morality entertained by a large class of females—aye, and men also, on this important question."[37]

Except for occasional condemnation of criminal abortionists, the AMA took no further formal action on abortion until 1967, when the Committee on Human Reproduction urged adoption of a policy in which the Association would oppose induced abortion except where (1) documented medical evidence showed a threat to the health or life of the mother; (2) the child may be born with incapacitating physical deformity or mental deficiency; or (3) a pregnancy resulting from legally established statutory or forcible rape or incest may constitute a threat to the physical or mental health of the patient. In addition, the committee proposed that two other physicians with recognized professional competency examine the patient and concur in writing as to the need for the abortion and that the physician perform the abortion in a hospital accredited by the Joint Commission on Accreditation of Hospitals. The AMA House of Delegates adopted this policy.[38] In 1970, the resolutions before the House of Delegates did not differ from the policy adopted in 1967 with the exception of the statement that "no party to the procedure should be requested to violate personally held moral principles."[39]

Scientific Context
Science, like religion, finds it difficult to establish the moment when life begins. One embryologist could define the unfertilized egg as a living entity but another embryologist could indicate great limitations in that definition because the unfertilized egg cannot continue to live more than a few days, has only half the chromosome supply that other body cells have, and therefore cannot develop without the addition of the sperm. This situation changes the moment an egg becomes impregnated by a male sperm, and this change results in a complete chromosome supply. The process of division begins and growth occurs rapidly; however, up to the sixth week of the embryo's existence, only an expert embryologist can tell whether the embryo is human or not. At the seventh week, human characteristics begin appearing, and by the 15th or 16th week the mother can feel the movements of the fetus.

All along the way of this remarkable process the embryo has what some call the marvelous gift of life, but others would argue that this is true only in the same sense that an animal or plant has life. The question remains as to when during this process this entity develops human life. No clear biological definition has been developed as to the beginning of human life. A larger question is whether physical life and personhood are the same things. Is it possible to have physical life and not have personhood?

Since the 1973 decision, advances in neonatal care have made 24 weeks the generally accepted time of viability. With this scientific change, the utility of the concept of viability for drawing legal and policy lines has been called into question.[40,41] The development of neonatal medicine, with its two billion dollar annual expenditures, allows for the treatment of imperiled or premature newborns who would have a few years ago died. This scientific development raises the question for the abortion debate of how we can ethically justify saving imperiled 22-

or 23-week-old newborns while accepting the abortion of perfectly healthy fetuses of the same age. The difference hangs on the notion of whether or not children are wanted. In the one case we speak of a cherished baby and in the other, a product of conception. Some public and health care professionals have difficulties with these distinctions.[42]

Social Context

In the years preceding the Supreme Court decision, dissatisfaction developed among physicians, legislators, judges, lawyers, and others regarding what they defined as the archaic abortion laws. Specifically, these dissatisfactions focused on (1) a decision for abortion based on and limited to maternal survival, whereas health and well-being received no consideration; (2) the complete failure to grant importance to the quality of the offspring; (3) no heed given to the circumstances under which impregnation occurred; and (4) the system under which abortion could be obtained invited inequities among those aborted.[43]

On one end of the abortion controversy, the group that wants more reform proposes that abortion should be a decision of the woman alone, or a decision made in consultation with her physician, and that the procedure should be performed in any public or private facility, with no legal statute imposing penalties on any party involved. This position assumes that no woman should bear any child she does not want, regardless of her reason, and that no legal statute or medical committee should interfere in her personal decision. The proponents of this position have used it to demonstrate how conservative the new abortion law is when judged by this group's position. In the argument for the woman's right to her personal decision about abortion, the only criterion is that the decision be consistent with the individual woman's personal set of moral and religious values, and in the final analysis only she can judge that.

Rossi believes that buried deeply beneath the abortion discussion one finds unresolved attitudes toward sex in this country. In addition, and perhaps compounding this situation, Americans seem to have a high tolerance for discrepancies between the moral norms they profess adherence to and what they privately practice and believe.[44] The National Opinion Research Center conducted a survey in 1965 asking a representative sample of 1484 adults in this country their views on the conditions under which a woman should be able to obtain a legal abortion. The major findings revealed widespread support among a majority of adults for legal abortion when a pregnancy involves a risk to maternal health, sexual assault, or probability of deformity in the fetus. The analysis of these data in terms of religious groups and sex difference showed that the important variable was not religion or sex per se, but the association of the two variables with church attendance. In other words, the more closely women and men, Catholic and Protestant, were involved with religion, the greater their tendency to reject a liberal stand on abortion.[45] A more recent study by Luker also reported this finding.[46]

The groups that believe that abortion can be morally justified do not wish to force women or health professionals who define it as morally wrong to participate in the procedure against their will. However, they do not wish to be denied the abortion choice, with the result of forcing women into childbearing against their will.[47] If women have access to abortion, the moral choice can be made; if society denies this access, however, the moral choice becomes determined for all by the values of some.

On the other end of the abortion controversy, we have the groups that would make abortion illegal and inaccessible, except perhaps under highly specified circumstances having to do with saving the mother's life. These groups have voiced two major concerns regarding the effects of liberalizing the abortion laws. The first concern has to do with the effect that undergoing an abortion will have on the individual woman, and the second has to do with the effects these laws will have on societal attitudes and behavior. As to the first concern, these groups assume that the more permissive the abortion laws, the more women will seek and, in fact, undergo abortion. This action denies the fetus whom they define as having personhood, the right to life. They argue that while giving the woman self-determination, easily accessible legal abortion does not afford the same right to the fetus, who cannot act in his own defense. The belief underlying this position places more weight on the benefit to society in keeping the legal presumption against abortion and less weight on the benefits to the prospective mother in being able to make her own decisions. One major component of this underlying belief focuses on the idea that destruction of the fetus, a human being, would diminish our reverence for life, our instinct for protecting the helpless, our concern that all forms of human life receive protection.[48] This position has little sociopsychological data with which to defend its position, and cross-cultural comparisons do not instruct us fully regarding our own situation. The antiabortion position and the proabortion position do, however, reflect the inherent strains in an irreducibly pluralist society and serve to bring into sharper focus the ethical dilemmas involved.

THE ETHICAL DILEMMA OF ABORTION

Since the 1973 Supreme Court decision, some believed that further ethical debate would only be academic in the most pejorative sense of that word. Others, however, believed that moral distinctions can be made within the framework of the reformed law and that these distinctions can assist the individual in developing or maintaining a moral position on abortion. The ethical dilemma involved can be limited to three of its dimensions for the purpose of discussion: (1) the rights of the fetus; (2) the rights and obligations of the mother; and (3) the rights and obligations of society. Two moral principles, consent and autonomy, are at the core of this ethical dilemma.

Rights of the Fetus

In presenting the *Roe v Wade* case before the Supreme Court, the lawyer argued that the Constitution does not define "person" in so many words. Although the 14th Amendment contains three references to "person," there can be no assurance that they have any prenatal application. The lawyer concluded that under the law, the unborn fetus is not a person. One important dimension of this ethical dilemma, however, asks for a definition of human life and some determination of when we can recognize its presence, so that we can then place a value on it and weigh it against other values. In the present state of biological ignorance on the matter and philosophical pluralism, the premise that the fetus is a person can be neither proved nor disproved to the satisfaction of all. Therefore, no one can assert superior moral sensitivity over opponents, and neither moral claim can rightfully eliminate the other from the political arena.[49]

Those concerned with what they consider a helpless minority, the unborn fetuses, judge the direct, intentional taking of innocent human life as an unacceptable means, however desirable the ends. Western religions, which teach an inclusive love of all people, foster a reverence for life and a respect for its sacredness that encourages an attitude of hesitancy toward the abortion act. The Protestant theologian Paul Ramsey found support in genetic research for the position that we should impute full human dignity to the nonviable fetus. Although not all ethicists would accept his moral reasoning, Ramsey argues that genetics tell us that we are what we become in every cell and attribute. Genetic data therefore provide us with a scientific approximation to the religious belief of ensoulment from conception.[50]

If we grant that from conception a fetus possesses humanity, we must then accord it all human rights, including the most basic one, the right to life. To kill that which possesses humanity is murder, except in the cases of war, self-defense, and capital punishment. Dealing with this, Bok's moral reasoning raises the larger question of whether the life of the fetus should receive the same protection as other lives. Basically, she asks the question: Is killing the fetus, by whatever means, and for whatever reasons, to be thought of as killing a human being? By drawing the line between abortions performed early in pregnancy and those done later, she develops the moral position that early abortions do not violate the principle of protection of life.[51]

One basic moral principle that has received much attention in recent years, that of informed consent, must be addressed in this dilemma. If one defines the fetus as possessing humanity at any point along the developmental continuum prior to birth, then the question must be asked: Who speaks for this human, using what criteria, and who guards his rights in this matter so vital to his existence? One argument, especially for the severely deformed fetus, says that if the fetus could speak for himself under these circumstances, he would consent to abortion. This argument can also be used to support abortions for the unwanted child without deformity. If the parent(s) does not want the child, what quality of life can the child expect to have? Will this child more likely become a victim of the increasing social problem, child abuse? The central question in this quality-of-life argument turns on the location of the line to be drawn. Will the line fall so as to include the variables of deformity, sex of the fetus, and the color of the hair and eyes as legitimate reasons for abortion?

Rights and Obligations of the Pregnant Woman

The other moral principle, autonomy, leads to the position that a woman has the right to her own body and the right to determine her own fertility. The dilemma arises out of the fact that the situation involves two lives. According to some, no one has an absolute, clear-cut right to control his or her fate where others share it. The Court took this consideration into account in its debate before changing the abortion law and when it made distinctions between what is allowed during the three trimesters as the embryo develops into a viable fetus.

Bok raises the question as to whether anyone, before or after birth, child or adult, has the right to continued dependence upon the bodily processes of another against the person's will.[52] Some argue that a woman, pregnant as a result of rape, incest, or in spite of every precaution, has no obligation to continue the pregnancy. In this case abortion is equated with cessation of continued support and not with unjust killing. An involuntarily pregnant woman can cease her support of life to the fetus without moral infringement of its right to life. Even those who support this argument under the circumstances specified might have difficulty using it in the situation of pregnancies entered into voluntarily. In this latter situation the obligation of the pregnant woman to the fetus could be defined differently and abortion might be considered a less responsible moral choice. Some take the position that pregnant women, no matter what the circumstances of conception, have obligations toward the life and well-being of the fetus that overshadow any discussion of the women's rights. In fact, in some discussions in certain political arenas the woman as a variable is not considered. The variables discussed are the father, the fetus, and the society. So we have a moral argument, where the stakes are high, in which some people support abortion on demand based on the woman's autonomy. At the same time we have people who oppose abortion perhaps except to save the life of the mother or not at all, based on the sanctity of life principle and the personhood of the fetus. To think in a simple way about this ethical dilemma, on the one hand the fetus is viewed as an object or thing while on the other, the woman is viewed as an object or thing. The political novel *The Handmaid's Tale* takes this woman-as-object idea and stretches it to a chilling conclusion.[53] In doing so, the darker interconnections between politics and sex are illuminated.

The exception to the argument for the overriding obligation to the fetus in the case of voluntary pregnancies may be, at least for some, the case involving an abnormal fetus. This raises the issue of quality of life not only for the yet unborn child, but also for the parents and for other children, if any, in the family.

Thompson in an earlier theoretical essay drew attention to the fact that the major focus in writings on abortion has been on what a third party, such as a physician, may or may not do when a woman requests an abortion. What the pregnant woman may do legally and morally was deduced from what third parties may do in the situation. Treating the matter of what the pregnant woman may do in such a fashion does not grant her the status of person that others insist on so firmly for the fetus. This comment finds grounding in the basic tenet of a democratic society that people must be permitted to exercise a maximum degree of individual freedom, bound only by a proper regard for the legitimate rights of other citizens.[54]

Little attention has been given to the role, rights, and obligations of the father in the abortion decision. That reflects the law's concern with the individual, in this case the pregnant woman.

Rights and Obligations of Society

One of the factors for any society in balancing values is the question of where to draw the line. In this case, that means under what conditions and considering the importance of what variables will society determine its abortion policy? If society develops a fairly restrictive policy, the argument could be made that some women would be threatened by the continuation of pregnancy, the new child would place great economic and psychological burdens on the family, the mode of existence and the career of some women would be seriously disrupted, and physically or mentally damaged infants would be born. On the other hand, if the policy permits women to obtain abortion with no restrictions or at least very limited restrictions, the "wedge" argument can be brought into the discussion. This argument says that there may be good reasons adduced for doing or not doing something because of what may possibly or predictably follow: What will come to be the case if our society does "X"? Will this social practice have consequences on other practices?

Applied to the abortion situation, the questions develop as follows: If social policy makes abortion available, will this lead that society to diminish its reverence for life and possibly to a lessening of its collective instinct for protecting the helpless? Would one such policy lead to other policies affecting the elderly, the mentally ill, and the mentally retarded? Could such policies push a society into disregarding the life of others who may not be productive or who may be a burden on society, such as the chronically ill or the chronically unemployed? No data from other countries with liberal abortion practices, such as Sweden and Japan, support this argument.

On a planet as interrelated as our own, some have taken the position that population control has become an overriding problem affecting every society and have suggested abortion as one method of dealing with this problem. Using demographic, economic, sociological, and psychological data, population experts have argued for and against abortion as an important means of birth control. One such expert has argued the issue from a moral perspective and on that basis has decided against abortion as a permissible means of population control.[55]

The crux of the question of abortion and the rights and obligations of society can be summarized in two questions. First, does society derive some benefits in legally and socially restricting abortion that override the benefits to the prospective mother of being able to make her own decisions? This question points out the need to balance the rights and obligations of society as a whole against the rights and obligations of the individual member of that society. Second, will the effects of our abortion policy be determined by the meaning that society attaches to abortion vis-à-vis its definition of human life per se and its definition of the quality of life derived? One of the major stresses surrounding the abortion issue is that if abortions are not available, those who define this procedure as right and good on the basis of their value system are denied access to abortion because of the value system of others who view it as wrong and bad. Some argue that, with the availability of abortions, no one forces another to undergo one against her own moral stand. The moral positions in any pluralistic society tend to reflect many diverse values, which can lead to intolerance of other viewpoints. The question of how we live with each other and each other's different values raises a central ethical dilemma.

Along with these central questions surrounding abortion, there have recently arisen other questions that demand attention. For example, the issue of minors seeking abortion has raised the question of the role of the parents in these cases. Should the parents be informed, and, if so, do they have the right to make the decision for their minor child? Does parental involvement extend to those minors deemed to be emancipated, such as those who support themselves, or to mature minors who are capable of making informed decisions about their own health and welfare?

Yet another issue that has developed in the abortion debate is whether the government should pay for abortion for poor women. When abortion is legal, is it just to deny the poor the same health services, including abortion, that others in the society have? Should we use tax monies for this purpose in a society where citizens are so deeply divided on the morality of abortion? It has been proposed to eliminate federal financing even in cases of incest or rape. Essentially, governmental funds would be available only to save the mother's life. Such questions as these, along with the major ethical questions of abortion itself, not only present us with personal ethical questions we need to think through, but, importantly for a democratic society, they have entered the arena of politics in such places as the United States Congress.

Another consideration that must be taken into account is allocation of resources. This dimension of the abortion dilemma has been brought into its sharpest focus by state governments denying public funds for abortion to women on welfare. What are the ethical implications of these decisions? All allocation of resources reflects values. That women who can afford to pay for abortions can legally have them while poor women cannot not only reflects some people's values regarding abortion but also reflects attitudes toward the poor.

Abortion is a societal issue that will not go away and, indeed, some argue that it should not go away. The central moral problems in the debate have remained remarkably stable over the years. The personhood argument says that either (1) the fetus lacks personhood and therefore is not entitled to protection against being killed; or (2) the fetus is a person and has this entitlement. The bodily support argument says that even if the personhood of the fetus were established, the choice of continuing the pregnancy belongs to the woman whose body is involved in that pregnancy. In the final analysis, how we understand ourselves as a people and how we define membership in this community is the larger concern for society.[56]

ABORTION AND NURSING

A brief review of the nursing and related literature provided insight into the activities and concerns of nurses as they have, in recent years, dealt with the ethical dilemmas of abortion. In 1967, the *American Journal of Nursing* (AJN) published a paper on abortion that pointed out that as society's views change, the law changes.[57] This reflected the ferment going on in the years just before the Supreme Court decision. At the American Nurses' Association (ANA) 1968 convention, the Division of Maternal and Child Health Nursing Practice presented a Statement to Study State Abortion Legislation. The delegates approved this statement with some discussion on whether the organization should take a stand on such a controversial issue that might be misunderstood. They expressed concern over the loose application of abortion laws that could result in serious risks to women and their families and expressed support of movements to examine and modify existing abortion laws.[58] At about the same time, an essay on nurses' attitudes and abortion addressed the issue of personal moral positions and professional obligations.[59] During the late 1960s and early 1970s, the AJN kept its readers abreast of the changes occurring in the state abortion laws in this country and of the changes and nurses' reactions to them in the United Kingdom. In addition, it reported the proceedings of an interdisciplinary panel on abortion.[60] Throughout the early 1970s, the AJN reported activities and experiences of individuals and groups concerned with abortion.[61-65] Occasionally, a paper presenting some aspect of nursing care and abortion appeared.[66,67] In January 1972, the *Journal* editor, Thelma Schorr, said in an editorial on abortion that "the search for moral values is part of what makes one human. Respecting the rights of others in their search also makes one humane."[68]

Over the past two decades, the research on nursing and abortion has focused, in the main, on attitudes. One study reported that in a sample of 500 nurses, 23 percent favored unrestricted abortion. Half or more favored abortion in cases of rape, defective fetus, physical or mental impairment of the woman, and grave economic hardship. Of the total, 75 percent stated that they would treat the abortion patient with as much understanding as any other patient.[69] Another study found older nurses and those at community hospitals less likely to condone abortion than their younger, university hospital counterparts.[70] A survey found that the kind and quality of involvement each health worker had had in dilemmas of unwanted pregnancy were important determinants of attitudes toward abortion. The organization and administration of abortion services and the social environment, including the attitude toward abortion in the general community and among professional peers, also affected the attitudes of health workers.[71] One year before the Court decision, research involving 50 nurses indicated that 22 did not favor a change in the law, for religious, ethical-professional, and social reasons.[72] A report sampling doctors and nurses who had actually participated in large numbers of abortions said that the doctors' involvement was perfunctory. Nursing personnel experienced considerable stress attempting to resolve their ambivalence about their participation in these procedures and reported some feelings of anxiety, depression, and anger toward patients for their sexual acting out.[73] When researchers compared the attitudes of social workers and nurses, they found that social workers evidenced more favorable attitudes toward abortion and explained the difference by the social structure of the two professions.[74] And finally, another study reported that significantly more nursing students and their faculty members opposed abortion on demand than did other health professionals and the general population with comparable education. Fewer nursing students and faculty members voiced willingness to help a client obtain an abortion than did other health professionals.[75]

In a philosophical analysis of ethical issues in refusing to provide patient care, the authors concluded that nurses may morally refuse a patient care assignment if, an only if, certain conditions are met. One such condition was refusal on religico-moral grounds when those objections have been made known in advance. No emergency can exist nor can the patient be placed in jeopardy by the refusal.[76] This condition would cover refusal to participate in the act of abortion itself. Whether it covers a refusal to care for the patient before or after the abortion is problematic in light of the ANA Code for Nurses, which states that nurses care for patients regardless of the patient's values and life-style.

If the nurse finds that because of her values she cannot condone abortion on any grounds, then the likelihood of her being able to care for an abortion patient without exhibiting unkind or even punitive behavior seems greatly diminished. In New York State, laws have been enacted that protect the individual who refuses to perform or participate in an abortion because this procedure is contrary to his or her conscience or religious beliefs. Such laws make the violation of this provision by an employer a misdemeanor. Furthermore, these laws indicate that no civil action for negligence or malpractice shall be maintained against a person refusing to perform or participate in an abortion. Every nurse confronted with this situation has both the right and the obligation to obtain information regarding state laws and institution policies on this matter.

A slightly more complicated situation may arise when a nurse approves of abortion for certain reasons but not for others, or when she believes abortion should be limited to the first trimester. Some nurses can work with patients admitted for a D and C procedure, since these abortions occur early in their pregnancies, while these same nurses find it difficult, if not impossible, to work with patients aborted by the saline method, since the fetuses will be further along in development. If the type of patients admitted match the nurse's category of permissible abortion, she should have no real ethical problems in providing nursing care; however, if they do not, she will need to work out a solution to her ethical dilemma in which her personal value system and her professional obligations conflict. A head nurse or nursing supervisor can play an important role here by discussing the issues with the staff nurse, provided her awareness of the ethical dilemma includes the balancing of the rights of the nurse-as-person with the obligations of the nurse-as-professional.

Perhaps the most worrisome type of situation arises with the nurse who either has given little thought to her moral position on abortion or in order to maintain her job denies to herself that she harbors resentment toward abortion patients. One can only hope that each nurse will seriously think about her beliefs on the sanctity of life and where she can morally draw the line between what she thinks is right or wrong, have some understanding of how she reached her conclusion, and realize how it will affect which functions she can or cannot perform because of this moral position.

In the last analysis, the nurse must arrive at a balance between her own values and her professional obligations to the patient. In the process of reasoning through the ethical dilemmas involved in abortion, the least that can be hoped is that she not abandon the patient. The most that can be hoped is that each nurse regard the rights of others as precious, as she would want her own regarded, and that within this context she view her obligations to herself, to the patient, to nursing, and to her place of employment.

It is difficult to find discussion of the abortion issue in recent nursing literature. As abortion has become an even more widely voiced issue at the national level, the position of nursing groups is difficult to determine. Perhaps this reflects the division on this issue found in society in general as much as anything else, or perhaps abortion as an ethical dilemma has not received the attention it deserves from the largest health care profession in the country. In California a survey conducted in late 1989 reported that 71 percent of the 500 nurses responding supported a woman's right to choose abortion. Twenty seven percent did not support a woman's right to choose abortion and 2 percent were undecided.[77] It is difficult to know the extent to which these findings can be generalized.

REFERENCES

1. Annas GJ: Webster and the politics of abortion. *Hastings Cent Rep* 19:36–38, March–April 1989.
2. LeBolt SA, Grimes DA, Cates W et al: Mortality from abortion and childbirth: Are the populations comparable? *JAMA* 248:188–191, July 9, 1982.
3. Crates W, Smith JC, Rochat RW, Grimes DA: Mortality from abortion and childbirth: Are the statistics biased? *JAMA* 248:192–196, July 9, 1982.
4. Cook RE, Hellegers AE, Hoyt RG, et al (eds): *The Terrible Choice: The Abortion Dilemma.* New York: Bantam; 1968: pp 40–41.
5. Guttmacher AF: Abortion—yesterday, today, and tomorrow. In Guttmacher AD (ed): *The Case for Legalized Abortion Now.* Berkeley, CA: Diablo; 1967: pp 8–9.
6. Tietze C, Lehfeldt H: Legal abortion in Eastern Europe. *JAMA* 175:1149–1154, 1961.
7. Tietze C: Abortion on request: Its consequences for population trends and public health. In Sloane RB (ed): *Abortion: Changing Views and Practice.* New York: Grune & Stratton; 1971: pp 165–166.

8. Gebhard PH, Pomeroy WB, Martin CE, et al: *Pregnancy, Birth and Abortion*. New York: Harper; 1958.
9. Rainwater L: *Family Design: Marital Sexuality, Family Size, and Contraception*. Chicago: Aldine; 1965.
10. Cartwright A: *Parents and Family Planning Service*. New York: Atherton; 1970.
11. Westoff LA, Westoff CF: *From Now to Zero*. Boston: Little, Brown; 1971.
12. Staples R: The sexuality of black women. *Sex Behav* 2:4–15, 1972.
13. Overstreet EW: California's abortion law—A second look. In Reiterman C (ed): *Abortion and the Unwanted Child*. New York: Springer; 1971: pp 15–26.
14. Smith KD, Steinhoff PG, Diamond M, et al: Abortion in Hawaii: The first 124 days. *Am J Public Health* 61:530–542, 1971.
15. Parker J, Nelson F: Abortion in New York City: The first nine months. *Fam Plann Perspect* 3:5–12, 1971.
16. Stone AA: The psychiatric dilemma. *Hum Sexuality* 4:29, 32, February 1970.
17. Pasnau: RO: *Medical Tribune*, August 4, 1971.
18. Blake J: Abortion and public opinion: The 1960-1970 decade. *Science* 171:540–549, 1971.
19. Lipson G, Wolman D: Polling Americans on birth control and population. *Fam Plann Perspect* 4:39–42, January 1972.
20. Callahan D: How technology is reframing the abortion debate. *Hastings Cent Rep*, 16:33–42, February 1986.
21. Bok, S: Ethics and decision making in medicine. Lecture at Harvard University, January 17, 1977.
22. Lappé M: How much do we want to know about the unborn? *Hastings Cent Rep*, 3:8–9, February 1973.
23. Castiglioni A: *A History of Medicine*. New York: Aronson; 1973.
24. Edlestein L: *The Hippocratic Oath: Text, Translation, and Interpretation*. Baltimore: Johns Hopkins University Press; 1967.
25. Noonan JT: An almost absolute value in history. In Noonan JT (ed): *The Morality of Abortion*. Cambridge, MA: Harvard University Press; 1970: p 4.
26. *Ibid.*, p 7.
27. Gustafson JM: A Protestant ethical approach. In Noonan JT (ed): *The Morality of Abortion*, p 116.
28. *Ibid.*, p 119.
29. Margolies IR: A Reform rabbi's view. In Hall RE (ed): *Abortion in a Changing World*. New York: Columbia University Press; 1970: pp 30–33.
30. Nazer IR: *Abortion in the Near East*. In Hall RE (ed): *Abortion in a Changing World* p 268.
31. Stern L: Abortion: Reform and the law. *J Crim Law* 59:84 1968.
32. Louisell DW, Noonan JT: Constitutional balance. In Noonan JT (ed): *The Morality of Abortion*, p 223.
33. Saltman J, Zimering S: *Abortion Today*. Springfield, Ill. Thomas, 1973, p 73.
34. Heller A, Whittington HG: The Colorado Story: Denver General Hospital experience with the change in the law on therapeutic abortion. *Am J Psychiatry* 125:809–816, 1968.
35. Cook RE, Hellegers AE, Hoyt RG, et al: *The Terrible Choice*, pp 60–61.
36. Johnsen D: A new threat to pregnant women's autonomy. *Hastings Cent Rep* 17:33–40, August 1987.
37. American Medical Association: *22 Transcript* 258:1871.

38. American Medical Association: *Proceedings of the House of Delegates,* June 1967, pp 40–51.
39. American Medical Association: *Proceedings of the House of Delegates,* June 1970, p 221.
40. Fost N, Chudwin D, Wilker D, et al: The limited moral significance of fetal viability. *Hastings Cent Rep* 10:13, December 1980.
41. Dunn PM, Stirrat GM: Capable of being born alive. *Lancet* 8376:553–554, March 10, 1984.
42. Callahan D: Technology, p 34.
43. Guttmacher AF: *Abortion—Yesterday,* p 12.
44. Rossi AS: Public views on abortion. In Guttmacher AF (ed): *Case for Legalized Abortion,* pp 31–33.
45. *Ibid.,* pp 35–51.
46. Luke K: *Abortion and the Politics of Motherhood.* Berkeley: University of California Press, 1984.
47. Pohlman E: Abortion dogmas needing research scrutiny. In Sloane RB: *Abortion,* p 17.
48. Cook RE, Hellegers AE, Hoyt RG, et al: *The Terrible Choice,* pp 65–66.
49. Cook RE, Hellegers AE, Hoyt RG, et al: *The Terrible Choice,* p 82.
50. Ramsey P: Points in deciding about abortion. In Noonan JT (ed): *The Morality of Abortion,* p 67.
51. Bok S: Ethical problems of abortion. *Hastings Cent Rep* 4:33–52, January 1974.
52. *Ibid.,* p 34.
53. Atwood M: *The Handmaid's Tale.* New York: Ballatine Books; 1987.
54. Thompson J: A defense of abortion. *Philos Public Policy,* Fall 1971, pp 47–66.
55. Dyck AJ: Is abortion necessary to solve population problems? In Hilgers TW, Horan DJ (eds): *Abortion and Social Justice.* New York: Sheed and Ward; 1972: pp 159–176.
56. Meilaender G: Abortion: The right to an argument. *Hastings Cent Rep* 19:13–16, November–December 1989.
57. Hershey N: As society's views change, laws change. *Am J Nurs* 67:2310–2312, November 1967.
58. ANA convention: A week of "firsts." *Am J Nurs* 68:1261, June 1968.
59. Fonseca JD: Induced abortion: Nursing attitudes and actions. *Am J Nurs* 68:1022–1027, May 1968.
60. Abortion. *Am J Nurs* 70:1919–1925, September 1970.
61. Nurses' feelings a problem under new abortion law. *Am J Nurs* 71:350, February 1971.
62. Catholic nurse-legislator files for abortion reform. *Am J Nurs* 71:459, March 1971.
63. Personal experience at a legal abortion center. *Am J Nurs* 72:110–112, January 1972.
64. Abortion yes or no; nurses organize both ways. *Am J Nurs* 72:416–418, March 1972.
65. Nurses' Association of American College of Obstetricians and Gynecologists: Principles and guidelines on abortion. *Am J Nurs* 72:1311, July 1972.
66. Cronewett LR, Choyce JM: Saline abortion. *Am J Nurs* 71:1754–1757, September 1971.

67. Ketter C, Copeland P: Counseling the abortion patient is more than talk. *Am J Nurs* 72:102–106, January 1972.
68. Schorr TM: Issues of conscience. *Am J Nurs* 72:61, January 1972.
69. What nurses think about abortion. *RN* June 1970, pp 40–43.
70. Brown NK, Thompson DJ, Bulger RJ, et al: How do nurses feel about euthanasia and abortion? *Am J Nurs* 71:1413–1416, July 1971.
71. Survey finds determinants of attitudes toward abortion. *Am J Nurs* 71:1900, October 1971.
72. Branson H: Nurses talk about abortion. *Am J Nurs* 72:106–109, Janaury 1972.
73. Kane FJ, Feldman M, Jain S, et al: Emotional reactions in abortion service personnel. *Arch Gen Psychiatry* 28:409–411, March 1973.
74. Hendershot GE, Grimm JW: Abortion attitudes among nurses and social workers. *Am J Public Health* 64:438–441, May 1974.
75. Rosen RAH, Werley HH, Ager JW, et al: Some organizational correlates to nursing students' attitudes toward abortion. *Nurs Res* 23:253–259, May-June 1974.
76. Brown JS, Davis AJ: Ethical issues in refusing to provide patient care. In Chask N (ed): *The Nursing Profession: Turning Points*. St. Louis: CV Mosby, 1990 pp 313–320.
77. Where do California nurses stand? *Calif Nurs Rev* 11:15, November–December 1989.

CHAPTER 9

Dying and Death

Issues surrounding dying and death raise many ethical concerns and questions for nurses as well as for the nursing profession. Many of these issues evoke our personal feelings of ambiguity about death. Indeed, some forms of dying while under nursing care challenge the prevalent view that death is the worst that can happen to us. Nurses provide care to patients throughout the life-span, from before birth to after death. Through the use of sophisticated life-support mechanisms and treatments, the process of dying is often prolonged in hospitals, nursing homes, or other institutions, where eight out of ten Americans die and where most nurses are still employed.[1] In the face of these statistics, it is not always clear that ethical principles such as "respect for persons," or "the noninfliction of harm" are being considered in practice.

Today we encounter troubling questions about when death actually occurs, the "quality of life," the "sanctity of life," verbal "do not resuscitate" orders, disclosure of terminal diagnoses to patients, and the individual's "right to die with dignity." There are other questions too. How should the interests of the individual patient, the family, health workers, and the community be weighed in making a decision about a congenitally deformed infant who will die without a sequence of surgical interventions and the use of costly medical resources? Who should decide? Does an individual have the right to "choose death"? Is there a moral difference between letting a person die and taking an action to hasten death? When, if ever, should life-sustaining treatment be withheld from patients who are unable to make this decision themselves? The implications of these questions are far-reaching and demand a thoughtful response from health care professionals, patients, families, the community, and society.

When the Quinlan case and decision in New Jersey (1976) were brought to public attention through the mass media, it served to refocus some of these questions for health professionals, for other professions (such as law and theology), and for the entire community. Another situation that also resulted in widespread ethical reflection involved the death of a newborn with Down's Syndrome and duodenal atresia at Johns Hopkins Hospital a few years earlier. The parents refused permission for surgery and the infant was allowed to die by starvation. Subsequently, the Joseph P. Kennedy, Jr. Foundation made a film that captured the pain and difficulty of the case. The many health professionals and students who have viewed the film have engaged in hours of agonizing discussion and moral questioning that the case elicits.[2] These and other situations poignantly illustrate the burdens placed on nurses and nursing by decisions made by others in the system but which nurses, nonetheless, are expected to implement. On the other hand, it is also in the areas of terminal illness and dying that nurses have made a difference in the options available to patients and their families, such as the development of hospice care, and in initiating changes in the decision-making process related to development of guidelines for orders not to resuscitate.

The ethical, legal, medical, social, cultural, psychological, and economic factors to be considered in near-death interventions (or decisions not to intervene) reflect individual, family, community, and professional values and must arbitrate between them. The numbers and kinds of factors, including values and clinical "facts," intersecting in each situation serve to further muddy the waters. The immediate decision is also often fraught with more distant implications, not the least of which includes those of social policy. But before we discuss end-of-life treatment, we would be well advised to reflect on the end of life per se.

DETERMINING WHEN SOMEONE IS DYING OR DEAD

According to *Webster's Third New International Dictionary, death* is "the ending of all vital functions without possibility of recovery: the end of life: the act, process, or fact of dying: the state of being no longer alive: a joyless, dull, tasteless existence: the state of being without full possession of enjoyment of the intellectual or physical faculties." When is an individual *dead*, with this tremendous range of ideas about death? This range implies the social, psychological, and physical dimensions of death. But which is determinative of death in the sense that one can say, "X" is dead? There is similar variability with use of the word *dead*. The definition ranges on a continuum from having ended existence as a living or growing thing, to being without power to move, feel, or respond, to being incapable of feeling or of being stirred emotionally or intellectually. Can one then be dead socially but not physically? This is a metaphysical question beyond the scope of this chapter. But both a process and an event are implied in these various notions.

Tolstoy's novel *The Death of Ivan Illyich* offers a telling description of the social, psychological, and physical aspects of death as a process for the individual and family. Again, these varied ideas of *death* and *dead* raise all the questions mentioned previously and increase the complexity for those who make decisions about whether or not respiratory support equipment should be discontinued or "extraordinary" measures begun for a particular individual.

Traditionally, it has been the physician who makes decisions concerning the dying patient. Fifty years ago, these decisions involved primarily the provision of comfort and reassurance for the patient and family. Today Morison talks about three possible areas of decision making for the physician. With the trend toward "death with dignity," the patient is or should also be involved in the choices of how to live while dying, the use of drugs to relieve pain, and the decision not to use medical measures that do not promote a cure. Morison discusses three areas of decision making. They are[3]:

1. Using all possible means, including "extraordinary" measures to keep the patient alive
2. Discontinuing "extraordinary" measures but continuing "ordinary" means
3. Taking some "positive" steps to hasten the individual's death

In making such decisions, one must take into account such factors as the determination of what is "extraordinary" or "burdensome," versus "ordinary" or "beneficial" in the treatment to be used for a particular patient, whether it be experimental drugs, complicated life-maintaining equipment, or even antibiotics. (It must be noted that though they are still commonly used in clinical settings, the terms "ordinary" and "extraordinary" have largely fallen into disuse among ethicists.) These decisions also raise moral questions about the factors that *ought to* figure in the decision-making process. For example, patients may be perceived as being more valuable to the living if they can be declared dead so that organs or tissues from their body can be used to benefit others. Some would see this as using one person primarily as a means to prolonging or improving another's life. In addition to factors already mentioned that may or may not enter into a decision of this nature, the "right to die" must also be taken into account. If one has the "right to life" at one end of the age spectrum, does one also have the "right to die" at the other end?

Criteria for the Determination of Brain Death

While the dictionary definitions of death give us clues about the process of death, they do not help in determining "the moment" of death. In contemporary health care, that moment is often obscured because of the use of ventilators, balloon pumps, or other life-sustaining technology.

Alternative means of determining death needed to be found. The most prominent effort to update the criteria for determination of death is found in the report of the Ad Hoc Committee of the Harvard Medical School, first issued in 1968.[4] This committee presented a set of criteria for determination of "brain death" as new criteria for judging biological death. This set has since become known as the "Harvard criteria" or the "Harvard definition" of death. The committee came up with several clinical criteria that were to be determinations made only by a physician. These determinations are summarized here as follows:[5]

1. Unreceptivity and unresponsivity, that is, intensely painful stimuli evoke no response
2. No movements or breathing, that is, observations are to be made for a period of at least one hour, and if the patient is on a respirator, the respirator may be turned off for 3 minutes to determine whether there is any effort at spontaneous breathing
3. No reflexes
4. Flat electroencephalogram (EEG) recorded for a minimum of 10 minutes and repeated at least 24 hours later with no change; the EEG is confirmatory only (i.e., not diagnostic)

These criteria are used as a means of determining that cardiopulmonary cessation has occurred when it cannot be otherwise measured because of technological interventions. Thus the criteria are used to establish that death, in our old familiar understanding, has occurred. These criteria do *not* establish a new definition of death; they are simply alternative means of measuring the same event—and they are considered to be invalid where hypothermia or evidence of drug intoxication exist.

The physician is to inform the patient's family, colleagues, and nurses who have been involved with the care of the patient when the determination of death has been made using the Harvard criteria. The committee emphasized that the patient should be declared dead before the respirator is turned off in order to provide physicians with a greater degree of legal protection.[5]

Issues concerning the determination of death clearly demonstrate the interaction of ethics and the law. Kansas has legislated a definition of death based on ordinary standards of medical practice, including loss of spontaneous brain function.[6] Some states have passed legislation that include brain death criteria. Both the Harvard criteria and the Kansas statute provide guidelines and a process for determining that biological death has occurred. In the Quinlan case, Judge Muir declared that physician decisions are overriding in the care of dying patients.[7] The decision still remains primarily with the physician, even though the Supreme Court of New Jersey modified the Muir decision to allow for such decisions to be made in consultation with an ethics committee.[8] The President's Commission for the Study of Ethical Problems in Medicine and Biomedical and Behavioral Research (the President's Commission) has developed uniform criteria for brain death to present to the states as a model for possible legislative action.

Morison raises questions about attempting to determine a specific time of death, since "life" in any organism, including humans, is not a clearly defined entity with sharp beginning and end points.[9] Issues of "life" are often clouded with those of "personhood" and "humanity." This is particularly evident in discussions of abortion. Morison sees the human organism as a complex interaction among individual cells, the totality of the cells, and the environment. The human system does not usually fail as a unit and so we may have to make clinical or ethical judgments about the value and intactness of the complex interactions of the organism; life is a continuous rather than a discontinuous process.

To some extent the process of dying is partially controlled today by individuals themselves in the choices they make about the use or refusal of available technologies or treatments. With this relative control over the time of death comes the necessity to think very carefully about who should be involved in decisions relating to this control and again what elements are important in the decision-making process.[9]

Kass does not think that Morison offers sufficient evidence for his view on the continuity of life and says, on the other hand, that the organism does die as a whole. According to Kass, there is still validity for the whole-body concept of death as an event and for using "reasonable criteria" for determining that a person has died.[10] These two viewpoints, presented only very briefly, again give the reader some notion of the complex philosophical, biological, and social issues involved in decisions made about death and the dying process.

To some extent, death can be delayed or prevented with the use of sophisticated technologies. Should these technologies be used simply because they are available? Should elderly comatose patients be taken from a nursing home to a renal dialysis center for thrice-weekly dialysis? A patient-centered ethic requires that the individual patient remain the center of decision making insofar as is possible, until a social consensus that would set boundaries on patient determination is otherwise reached. All of these issues and questions seem to pivot on questions about the quality of life when dying is prolonged through medical and nursing intervention. Discussions of active euthanasia nip at the heels of discussions of the quality of life when dying is prolonged through the use of technology.

EUTHANASIA AND THE WITHHOLDING OR WITHDRAWAL OF TREATMENT

The concept of *euthanasia* comes from the Greek, meaning good or pleasant death. Is death ever preferable to life? Is there a moral difference between "letting die" and "hastening death," in light of the moral law that "thou shalt not kill?" At present, there is mixed agreement on answers to these questions. One needs to consider carefully what the best interests are for a particular patient in a specific situation and to distinguish this from the interests of the provider, institution, and society. The following discussion focuses primarily on the dying adult patient and on ethical (as distinct from religious) considerations per se.

In attempting to provide at least tentative solutions to the initial question, Bok suggests an examination of the following criteria for decision making as a first step.[11]

1. Who decides? The physician, guardian, patient, family member, clergyman, or a committee?
2. For whom does one decide? Oneself, one for whom one is acting as a proxy, or others?
3. What additional criteria are used (e.g., psychological, economic, social) after the medical status of the patient has been established?
4. What degree of consent is required of the patient?

Decision making should also consider the moral principles involved, such as respect for autonomy, the obligation to do no harm, and the requirement to tell the truth. Are they being affirmed or negated by particular alternatives proposed? In considering question 4 above, Bok states that euthanasia should be considered only in relation to those who can ask to die (what is commonly called "voluntary" euthanasia). This position eliminates newborns and infants from its consideration.[12] It is also problematical in that it excludes as well those individuals "kept alive" on machines who are unable to participate in decision making.

Duff, Campbell, and Shaw, physicians, and McCormick, a theologian, take another position on decision making for newborns and argue that in certain circumstances, some severely deformed newborns should be allowed to die by withdrawing or withholding treatment. These authors feel that these decisions should be made by parents with the assistance of professional advisors, usually physicians, since the parents are the most familiar with the human complexities of a given situation.[13-15] In recent years, when parental decisions for nontreatment of infants have been brought to the courts, most court decisions have required that treatment be given. These decisions make it clear that there is a general legal duty to treat a child. The reader is already aware of other views mentioned in the earlier section on determining when a person is dying or dead. These opposing views reflect the complexity and conflict that exist when we attempt to answer the questions surrounding dying and death.

To look further at questions related to euthanasia, there is a continuum of intervention for decision makers ranging from an anti-euthanasia absolutist position on the sanctity of life, to an equally absolutist pro-euthanasia view based on some determination of an inadequate quality of life, or on a supposed absolute right to decide. The absolutist anti-euthanasia position commits one to vigorous treatment to preserve life at any or all costs and is not in accord with general understanding of the sanctity of life principle. More moderate positions require the use of nonburdensome treatments without necessarily requiring the use of "heroic measures." There is difficulty in determining exactly what constitutes (and who decides what constitutes) burdensomeness. If we follow the general norm that the patient's decisions are determinative about her or his own care, what constitutes burdensomeness becomes particularly difficult when the patient cannot express the degree of burden that he or she feels.

One author has defined *ordinary* (or *nonburdensome*) means of preserving life as including all medicines, treatments, and surgical procedures that offer *reasonable hope of benefit* to a patient and can be obtained and used *without excessive pain, expense or other inconveniences. Extraordinary* (or *burdensome*) means are those that are very costly, unusual, difficult, or dangerous, or do *not* offer a reasonable hope of benefit to the patient at a given time and place.[16] These determinations may differ in a large teaching hospital from the ones made in a small community hospital or in the particular setting where the dying individual is placed. What may be considered ordinary or nonburdensome treatment to or for one patient may be considered extraordinary or burdensome to or for another, for example the use of antibiotics for a patient with pneumonia only as opposed to their use for the patient who has terminal cancer with metastases to the brain and liver who develops pneumonia.

Some regard withdrawal of treatment to let the patient die as a form of passive euthanasia, while others maintain that it is the intent (i.e., that the patient's death is intended) rather than the withdrawal of treatment itself that determines whether or not euthanasia is involved. In "letting die, "treatment is withheld or ongoing treatment withdrawn with or without the consent of the patient.[17] The withdrawal of treatment to allow a patient to die is still a morally controversial topic for many health professionals even though it has received ample attention in the ethical literature, to the point of being considered a "settled question," as we shall see in a moment.

Active euthanasia is considered to include such actions as giving patients the means to kill themselves ("assisted suicide") or directly bringing about the patient's death with or without consent, for instance through the lethal injection of potassium chloride.[18]

Where does the "right" of patients to control their own dying fit into this consideration of euthanasia? Do individuals have the "right to die," or even to kill themselves in a hospital committed to preserving life? Can a patient refuse life-saving treatment? Some have said that institutional inhumanity is the enemy, not death *per se*.[19]

According to Simons, a Florida attorney, there is no provision in the law that compels a competent person to seek medical care, except when the illness is a threat to the public health or safety—for example, with a communicable disease. In the case of *Palm Springs General Hospital, Inc. v Martinez*, the hospital and the attending physician were not required to perform surgery or transfusions against the patient's will.[20] There have been contradictory findings in various cases in which individuals refused life-saving blood transfusions because of religious beliefs—for example, the case of *Kennedy Memorial Hospital v Heston*, in which it was said that the hospital ethics required life-saving treatment.[21] In *Erickson v Dilgard*, on the other hand, it was found that the patient did have the right to refuse blood transfusion even though he would most likely die without it.[22] In 1977, the Massachusetts Supreme Court decided in the Saikewicz case that the courts should most appropriately make decisions about nontreatment for those incompetent to make their own decisions. This court also affirmed that all patients have the right to refuse life-sustaining treatment that will not cure or preserve life.

In the Karen Quinlan case, Judge Muir said that when an adult is rendered incompetent, society expects that the attending physician's decision will prevail even when there is a conflict with a family decision. The Quinlan decision also supported a role for ethics committees in the decision-making process (though this concept of an ethics committee is what would more commonly be regarded as a prognosis committee). Judge Muir's decision conflicts with that of a national public opinion poll. When asked about a patient dying in the hospital with no hope of cure, over 50% of the sample said that is was all right to let the person die and that the decision should be made by family members or by the physician in conjunction with family members. Only 7% felt that it was the decision of the patient's physician alone. Physicians seem to agree with the public rather than with Judge Muir. In 1973, the American Medical Association (AMA) House of Delegates adopted a statement that condemned physicians agreeing to perform "mercy killing" (active euthanasia) but said that stopping extraordinary means to prolong biological life is the decision of the patient or his immediate family, with freely available advice and the judgment of the physician.[23] A general social consensus seems to be developing that physicians should not be the only individuals to make decisions related to prolonging life or hastening death.

In the early 1980s, the President appointed a commission to investigate several major ethical issues. That commission was formally named the President' Commission for the Study of Ethical Problems in Medicine and Biomedical and Behavioral Research. Of the reports that it issued, the one entitled *Deciding to Forego Life-Sustaining Treatment* is of special importance to the discussion here. In that report, the President's Commission maintained that:

> Nothing in current law precludes ethically sound decision making. Neither criminal nor civil law—if properly interpreted and applied . . . forces patients to undergo procedures that will increase their suffering when they wish to avoid this by foregoing life-sustaining treatment.*

The commission further held that

> The distinction between failing to initiate and stopping therapy—that is, withholding versus withdrawing treatment—is not itself of moral [or legal] importance. A justification that is adequate for not commencing a treatment is also sufficient for ceasing it.**

Life-sustaining or death-prolonging treatment may be withheld or may be withdrawn when it is against the patient's wishes, providing that the patient is fully informed and freely consenting; it may also be withheld or withdrawn when it will or has begun to harm the patient, or when it is not benefitting the patient or will not.

Thus, for the most part, ethicists have agreed that when life-sustaining treatment will constitute the violation of the patient's dignity, humanity, well-being, or integrity, it need not be given or continued. This has become a "settled" issue. The one area of concern that has yet to be resolved is the administration of food and fluid, particularly by "medical means."

The Cruzan case has recently brought ethical issues surrounding this specific form of treatment into the public arena. Nancy Cruzan, a 32-year-old woman, was tragically rendered in a persistent vegetative state as the result of an auto accident 6 years ago. Before the accident, Cruzan had made a number of statements that she would never wish to live as a "vegetable" and that she did not view death as the worst possible thing that could happen to her. Thus in accord with what they knew to be her wishes and on the basis of her former life-style and personality, her parents, who are also her legal guardians, sought to have Cruzan's gastrostomy tube removed so that she might be allowed to die.

The Supreme Court of the state of Missouri refused to allow the removal of the gastrostomy tube. This decision flew in the face of the

---

*President's Commission for the Study of Ethical Problems in Medicine and Biomedical and Behavioral Research. *Deciding to Forego Life-Sustaining Treatment*; March 1983, p 89.
**Ibid, p 61.

trend of the law and ethics and many previous court precedents regarding withdrawal of treatment. The court decision is lengthy and poorly argued, but it essentially held that the state had a compelling interest in preserving life. It did not matter that Cruzan would not emerge from the persistent vegetative state, nor that she had stated to her parents and others that she would never have wanted treatment under the conditions to which she was subject. The court, instead, demanded "clear proof" of Cruzan's position—such as a written statement to that effect. This case was argued before the Supreme Court of the United States on December 6, 1989. The 1990 decision of the Supreme Court has profound implications for how the issue of nutrition and hydration is approached in clinical practice, particularly in terms of whether such treatment may be withdrawn in accord with the patient or family wishes and patients be allowed to die. A constitutional right to refuse life-preserving medical therapy is recognized, while allowing states to develop procedures for determination of patient intent.

In using the term *euthanasia*, some authors make a distinction between mercy killing and allowing people to die. They claim that one is an act of commission, the other an act of omission. A further distinction is made between voluntary (with patient permission) and involuntary (without patient permission) euthanasia. Others consider euthanasia to be any act done by another that results in *intentionally* bringing about death, whether it is by an act of omission or commission, but that treatment withdrawal without intent to bring about death does not constitute euthanasia. It has also been argued that there is no moral distinction between active and passive euthanasia because the end result, death of the patient, is the same. Acts of omission are seen as not interfering with the natural process of dying, while euthanasia-as-mercy-killing is seen as inducing death (as in the AMA House of Delegates' statement). Another distinction is that the "right to die" is associated only with the individual, whereas euthanasia demands that someone else, or society, intervene to induce or to assist in inducing death. This raises the question as to whether society or any of its members should accept such an obligation.[24]

In the United States, there are some serious gaps in the law for dealing with the broad issue of euthanasia. Euthanasia is still regarded as a form of homicide; patient consent or request for euthanasia is not legally acceptable as a defense. The law does, however, take into account whether the situation involves an act or a failure to act; to some extent, the law does make a distinction between active and passive euthanasia. According to Fletcher, there is no case in the Anglo-American tradition of law in which a physician has been convicted of murder or manslaughter for having committed a passive act to end the suffering of a patient.[25] This tradition, then, seems to consider the intent of the physician. Nevertheless, uncertainty still exists as to the legal consequences that may result for the health professional.

There are different ethical points of view on euthanasia that are significant to the nurse, other health professionals, and society in seeking to articulate a moral position on euthanasia. One position, sometimes called the "new morality," supports a value system that puts humanness, human dignity, and personal integrity above biological life and functions. This position arises from the ancient religious belief that the core of humanness lies in the rational faculty, that is, in one's ability or potential to be rational. What counts as ethically right action is whether or not human needs come first. The moral defense is that euthanasia reduces suffering and helps the patient die rather than prolonging a slow, ugly, dehumanizing death. This position holds the value that death is not the worst thing that can happen to an individual. Both Eastern and Western religious traditions agree that one is not morally obligated to preserve life in all cases. A second position, the Roman Catholic position, as represented in the Pope's position as long ago as 1957, is that it is not necessary to use "extraordinary" means to prolong life for the terminally ill person.[26]

One objection to the general idea of euthanasia is that the same thing will happen as happened in Nazi Germany; this is a kind of "wedge" argument. Kohl sees this particular wedge argument as claiming that if beneficent euthanasia, a kindly act, can be morally justified, then euthanasia for other purposes may be practiced and justified.[27] This kind of thinking ignores the fact that the Nazis engaged in genocide and killing for experimental purposes, *not* "mercy killing" in the sense of a merciful act of kindness.

On the other hand, one should not ignore the findings of research in which, for example, a sample of university students was asked a variety of questions related to euthanasia and a "final solution" to problems of overpopulation and misery. Over half of the respondents said that society should get rid of "unfit" persons as a "final solution."[28] Fletcher feels that it is still more difficult to morally justify letting someone die a slow, dehumanized death than not letting him do so.[29] For Fletcher, the practice of euthanasia-as-merciful-killing implies compassion on the part of the agent and society. Others do not agree, because killing for them always has evil characteristics, even when killing is in self-defense.

In considering whether or not suffering justifies killing, the principle of "proportionate good" may be used. This is the principle of balancing the benefits and harms of an action for the suffering individual. A reminder of the Rawlsian criterion for moral principles follows, to be used in deciding whether or not one can morally justify the "proportionate good" principles for any form of euthanasia. A moral principle should be[30]:

1. *General* in the sense that it expresses general properties and relationships and is not specific to individual persons or relationships

2. *Universal* in the sense that it applies to everyone and is chosen with a view of the consequences if everyone complies
3. *Public* in the sense that everyone knows and recognizes the principle as operative in society
4. An *imposition of order* on conflicting claims in terms of using justice and right to make the adjustment rather than the capacity to coerce
5. *Final* in the sense that this is the last court of appeal and overrides law, custom, social rules, and self-interest

One may question whether the "proportionate good" principle meets all these criteria in relation to the question of active euthanasia. One could say that this principle is in line with a "quality of life" ethic, which says that some lives are not worth living. In other words, death is not the worst thing that can happen to a person.

Dyck argues against euthanasia by arguing for an "ethic of bene-mortasia," which comes from the Latin, meaning a good or kind death. This is an ethic of obligation and is concerned with how we should behave toward those who are dying or whose death appears to be a merciful event. Mercy is considered to be a moral obligation in this position. In the face of continuing debate by proponents of beneficent euthanasia and opponents of it, the ethic of benemortasia suggests the following kinds of care for patients who are considered to be "imminently dying"[31]:

1. The relief of pain
2. The relief of suffering
3. Respect for the right of an individual to refuse treatment
4. Universal provision of health care in the sense that individuals and families would not have to bear alone the burden of catastrophic medical care

A third position on euthanasia as "mercy killing" states that mercy killing as active euthanasia is never permissible and that respectful treatment of patients as persons is the fundamental principle of medical ethics. This position does make a moral distinction between killing and allowing to die. Disease is accepted as a cause of death, but a human agent should not be the cause of death, according to this position. This seems to actually rule out both active and passive euthanasia. Another distinction that could be made is between not actively fighting death and actively putting an end to life. A further argument is that the starting point for considering the morality of any kind of killing is that evil is always present in the act of killing.

This third position holds that the physical cannot be separated and excluded from what makes a person a person. A person is not just cerebral function. How does one determine what is "a person" for decision-making purposes? Weber says that the sanctity of life ethic should not be put aside in favor of a quality of life ethic, as this will weaken man's respect for man and presents a dehumanizing ethic dangerous to human community.[32] This fear and other objections are expressed by various authors in considering whether and what kind of legislation should be enacted in this area.[33-35] What is best for the individual? What is best for society, now and in the future? These interests conflict in the euthanasia issue.

Weber goes on to say in the third view that there does come a time to cease prolonging life and to concentrate on the needs of the dying person in an attempt to provide a peaceful death for the overall good of the individual patient. He warns, however, that the physician must be aware that what is considered to be the medical good of the patient is not always what the patient wants.[36] What the patient wants may change over time, making decisions even more slippery, leaving the professional to mistakes of interpretation.[37] A further complication is that the physician may have developed an ethic, which claims that it is a physician's duty to preserve life as long as possible. Consequences to the patient are not considered as important as the physician's hope to avoid criticism for stopping life-support mechanisms prematurely.[38] So there are patients who are dead by the brain death criteria but are still kept biologically "alive" by technological means.

Decisions Not to Resuscitate and Advance Directives

In discussing the decision not to resuscitate, Weber says that it is fully compatible with respect for the intrinsic value of human life. He views the decision not to resuscitate under specific circumstances as a refusal to attempt to control life and death any further through the use of technology.[39] Two hospitals in the Boston area reported on their efforts to develop guidelines for making the decision not to reuscitate.[40,41] The Minnesota Medical Association also approved Do Not Resuscitate (DNR) Guidelines in 1981.

Further efforts to clarify the position of individuals and society on the right to die with dignity are seen in the development of living wills by individuals and groups, including a group called Concern for Dying: An Educational Council.[42] The living will prepared by Concern for Dying (formerly the Euthanasia Educational Council) has been used as a model for "death with dignity" bills introduced into state legislatures. One example, which appeared in an article by Sisela Bok, is presented here[43]:

DIRECTIONS FOR MY CARE*

I, _____, want to participate in my own medical care as long as I am able. But I recognize that an accident or illness may someday

*Reprinted by permission. From the New England Journal of Medicine (295:367–369, 1976)

make me unable to do so. Should this come to be the case, this document is intended to direct those who make choices on my behalf. I have prepared it while still legally competent and of sound mind. If these instructions create a conflict with the desires of my relatives, or with hospital policies or with the principles of those providing care, I ask that my instructions prevail, unless they are contrary to existing law or would expose medical personnel or the hospital to a substantial risk of legal liability.

I wish to live a full and long life, but not at all costs. If my death is near and cannot be avoided, and if I have lost the ability to interact with others and have no reasonable chance of regaining this ability, or if my suffering is intense and irreversible, I do not want to have my life prolonged. I would then ask not to be subjected to surgery or resuscitation. Nor would I then wish to have life support from mechanical ventilators, intensive care services, or other life-prolonging procedures, including the administration of antibiotics and blood products. I would wish, rather, to have care which brings comfort and support, which facilitates my interaction with others to the extent that this is possible, and which brings peace.

In order to carry out these instructions and to interpret them, I authorize _____ to accept, plan, and refuse treatment on my behalf in cooperation with attending physicians and health personnel. This person knows how I value the experience of living, and how I would weigh incompetence, suffering, and dying.

Should it be impossible to reach this person, I authorize _____ to make such choices for me. I have discussed my desires concerning terminal care with them, and I trust their judgment on my behalf.

In addition, I have discussed the following specific instructions regarding my care:
(Please continue on back)
Date _____ Signed _____

Witnessed by _____ and by_____

Bok suggests that each individual try to write a living will in order to gain some understanding of the complexities of doing this.[43] One problem often raised in relation to living wills is that individuals may feel differently at the time of writing the will from the way they do later when they become ill. People can change their minds at any time and destroy a living will document. This problem can also be modified by sharing one's wishes with family members and one's physician whenever possible.

The Natural Death Act (1976) in California (its "living will" legislation) recognizes the rights of adults to prepare written instructions authorizing their physicians to withhold or withdraw life-sustaining procedures in specified circumstances of terminal illness. A major purpose of the original bill was to settle a number of legal issues concerned with professional liability and insurance coverage. This Act relieves physicians, health facilities, and other licensed health professionals of civil liability for carrying out directives as defined in the bill. The bill declares that death resulting from carrying out a directive does not constitute suicide, thus resolving this issue in relation to insurance policies, as well.[44] Although this legislation provides answers and guidelines for some problems, it has always been recognized that public policy of this import will raise a host of additional issues in relation to interpretation.

In addition to living will or legislation for advance directives a number of states have provisions for designating a "durable power of attorney for health care" (DPHC). Though the legislation varies from state to state, the DPHC allows adults to designate another (and an alternate) as decision maker for health care decisions when the person cannot make their own decisions. Such documents allow for the power of attorney to be given to any adult, including a non-family member. While the DPHC is not a living will, some forms allow the person to specifiy the sorts of treatments that would or would not be acceptable at the end of life. For the person who holds the power of attorney (emphasis is on *power*; the person need not be a lawyer) his or her decisions have the force of the patient's own decisions and cannot be challenged unless they appear to be clearly contrary to the patient's own wishes.

End-of-Life Treatment Decisions and the Pediatric Patient

Previous discussion of the problem of active euthanasia and passive euthanasia as "allowing to die" focused primarily on adult and elderly patients. These issues were mentioned only briefly in relation to severely deformed newborns and children with terminal illness. Many of the same issues and questions involving adults apply to children and newborns. One basic issue when children and infants are involved concerns who should make what decisions. The physician? The parents? The child? One concern is whether or not a society should even consider the nontreatment option for children. What are the implications for individuals and the human community, again, in terms of the value of life? Some see this as a question of infanticide, others see it as a "quality of life" issue.[45-49] Englehardt sees other special concerns arising in relation to euthanasia and young children—for example, the legal standing of the rights of children, the status of parental rights, and the obligations of adults to prevent suffering in children.[50] All these concerns are still raised whenever severely deformed infants and terminally ill children receive care. What are ordinary and extraordinary measures in a newborn intensive care unit? Do they depend on the locally available technology? Do health professionals have obligations to always use the technology available without looking at how lives are affected by it now and in the foreseeable future?

In a discussion of nontreatment of newborns with birth defects, Robertson, a lawyer, argues that the "current haphazard, arbitrary patterns of selection for nontreatment" will probably continue unless substantive and procedural criteria are developed as guidelines for decision making in this area that is full of stress and pain. He suggests guidelines that would identify those situations in which treatment would invariably be required, such as low-lesion spina bifida; those situations in which treatment could invariably be withheld, such as with anencephaly; and those cases in which the situation is less clear and decisions depend on the facts of the individual case.[51]

In summary, this brief overview of some of the issues and complexities of decision making related to euthanasia, death, and dying does not provide us with any readymade answers. What it does do is give the reader some idea of directions taken by individuals, institutions, and society in seeking ways to make more ethically appropriate decisions in this area.

SUICIDE AS AN ETHICAL DILEMMA

Suicide is the 10th leading cause of death in the United States, causing approximately 25,000 deaths per year. Annual attempts at suicide may range as high as 400,000.[52] Suicide has been seen variously as an affirmation of life, a denial of life, and a questioning of life. The traditional religious teachings of the Western religions have condemned all intentional acts of self-destruction.[53] Though it is all too simple a reduction of their position, one might say that traditionally Western theologies have regarded life as a gift of God, belonging to God, but given to humankind for its stewardship. Suicide, then, has been seen as a usurpation of God's authority and thus as sin, because it involves the claim that one's life is one's own (and not belonging to God) to do with as one pleases.

According to the philosopher Kant, who was concerned to separate religion and ethics, humans rightfully do not have the power of disposal of their own bodies. One can only treat one's body as one chooses in relation to self-preservation.[54] These views are being challenged in today's society, as they always have been. Realizing that suicide often occurs when a person is despondent or under duress, and thus less than fully voluntary, the Act of 1961 declared that suicide should no longer be regarded as a criminal act.[55]

Talking about the right to commit suicide, Murphy, a psychiatrist, says that "rational" suicide may be ascribed to those persons suffering from a terminal disease. However, the majority of persons who commit suicide are not terminally ill. The majority suffer from clinically recognizable psychiatric illnesses and have sought help from physicians. Only a few have received necessary treatment.[56] Some light is thrown on this by a study done in the early 1970s that found that 75 percent of all suicide victims consulted a physician before their act. Another finding was that the physician respondents had inadequate knowledge of suicide. The majority did not know the most vulnerable age group and many had negative attitudes toward suicide and people who attempt it.[57]

Heifetz, a neurosurgeon, states that under certain circumstances the people who are severely ill, near death, and who wish to commit suicide should receive help from their physicians. Laws exist in Uruguay, Switzerland, Peru, Japan, and Germany, but not the United States, for such assistance by the physician. However, Heifetz points out that this group must be considered separately from the lonely, the elderly, and the physically handicapped who may also seek to commit suicide and ask another's assistance.[58]

The question of the individual's right to self-determination is a basic consideration in talking about the ethical dimensions of suicide. There are positions on both ends of the continuum. They range from the position that the individuals have the right to self-determination and that they should retain this right even if they are considered by some to be potentially dangerous or suicidal, to the view that the physician has the obligation to support "the desire for life" that exists even in those who feel that this desire has left them, for example, individuals suffering from depression.[59,60] Other major arguments against suicide are that it is a crime against society, a cowardly act, a violation of one's duty to God, unnatural, and an insult to human dignity, and that it is cruel because it inflicts pain upon one's family and friends. Hook suggests that this last argument that considers consequences, while not absolute, has greater weight than any of the previous arguments.[61]

Arguments have been made that suicide may be ethically justifiable under certain conditions. One such argument is that no rational morality would require that certain lives be continued in the face of disastrous accidents of birth or of illnesses for which there are not effective remedial measures. Another argument is that no social morality can be equally binding on everyone in society unless there is more equality in distributing the necessities, sometimes called the goods, of life.[62] One thinks in terms of justice as fairness and the more equal distribution of society's benefits and harms. The obligation to provide a just society in which all can live well seems to rest with those who say that one should not commit suicide.

In summary, the question of suicide is still controversial in our society and raises many profound ethical questions for the health professional about the individual's right to self-determination vis-à-vis the right of the human community to preserve itself.

FURTHER THOUGHTS FOR NURSING PRACTICE

Much of the nursing literature has focused primarily on attitudes toward death and dying patients; the depersonalized, institutionalized dying process; and the nurse's personal experiences with dying patients and their families.[63-71] Little has been written on the ethical dilemmas faced by nurses in relation to the dying patient, the family, and other health professionals, particularly the physician. This is changing, particularly in relation to verbal "no code" orders and the development of hospice care.

Nurses should examine, individually and collectively, their own values in relation to death, quality of life, the importance of the individual needs of patients, and such moral principles as self-determination for the dying patient, on the bases of respect for the person, the obligation to do no harm, and distributive justice.

Hershey, a lawyer, says that the nurse's *legal* responsibility is to respect the medical decision.[72] One issue, however, that frequently arises for nurses is that they do not always have written orders on which to rely. Decisions will be made by nurses for specific patients if they have a cardiac arrest and only verbal "no code" orders exist. It is generally understood that if there are no written orders for "no code" and a patient arrests, the nurse must "code" the patient.

One example of hospital efforts to recognize a patient's right to refuse available medical procedures, in light of the hospital's primary philosophy to preserve life, is the development of guidelines for orders not to resuscitate. According to these guidelines, physicians have the primary obligation to explore the implications of this decision with the patient and family, but the initial judgment should be discussed first with the other physicians, nurses, and any others directly involved with the patient's care. This provides an opportunity for nurses to add their observations and assessment of a patient to those of others in the decision-making process and to carry out the *caring* process for dying patients. It is the responsibility of the physician not only to actually record the order not to resuscitate but to convey the meaning of this order for a particular patient to medical, nursing, and other appropriate staff members.[73] Nurses are in a key position to notify the physician if the patient's condition changes, which change would indicate that the orders may need reassessment.

Nurses are involved in the emotional support needed by the patient's family as they are often the most constant resource for families. Various authors discuss how nurses can be most helpful to families of dying patients.[74,75] Research has identified some specific needs of spouses of dying patients.[77] These needs are to be with the dying person, to be helpful to the dying person, to be assured of the comfort of the dying person, to be informed of the mate's condition, to be informed of impending death, to be able to air emotions, to have the comfort and support of other family members, and to have acceptance, support, and comfort from health professionals. Half of the study sample reported that they did not have this last need met. Spouses generally agreed that nurses had been helpful to their dying mates but were perceived as being too busy to help the families. Nurses can be facilitators for meeting most of these needs, even in intensive care settings, by making themselves available to families. This is not without strain and tension for the nurses.[77,78] The next question is whether nursing administration has a moral obligation to provide support systems for nursing staff members involved with critically ill and dying patients. Some institutions already provide such support for nurses and physicians. Nurses can also initiate collaborative efforts with others, such as chaplains and social workers, to meet the needs of families of dying patients.

Another issue facing nurses in many hospitals concerns the patient who arrives on the unit with a "living will," or advance directive, attached to the chart in one of the states where these documents are not legally binding. This may present a conflict between respect for patient autonomy and authority and that of the physician. This is one example of an issue in which an interdisciplinary committee constituted at the institutional level to discuss ethical issues in patient care could be most helpful.[79] Nursing can and should actively participate in these groups, as they are a primary resource to their patients and because they confront so many of these issues in their daily practice.

Smith says that such committees, when discussing issues of care for the dying, often fall into two categories: those with the "participant" point of view and those with the "administrative" perspective. Nurses and physicians are usually in the first group—that is, they often identify with the patient and what they assume to be in the best interests of the patient. The second perspective views the dying patient as a managerial problem and is more concerned with such issues as the use of hospital resources. Problems are implicit in these two viewpoints. The "participant" perspective in advocating death with dignity and the rights of patients to refuse treatment often ignores consideration of when and under what conditions patients might choose death. Health professionals must also guard against imposing their own values on patients and families. The "administrative" viewpoint, frequently a more utilitarian view, is concerned with efficient use of resources and the equality of treatment for all patients, thus ignoring the diversity of individual patient needs.[80]

Ramsey warns that in disagreements between these viewpoints, questions should be resolved as *patient* policy questions, not as hospital or public policy questions, such as those concerning limited beds or other limited hospital resources.[81] The danger exists that more and more decisions will be made on the basis of economic considerations and needs that can be accommodated or on a utilitarian ethic that considers the greatest happiness for the greatest number as the determinant in decision making. In light of this, one needs to refocus on the moral principles of "doing no harm," justice as equal treatment, and respect for values of patients and families, with both common and individual needs considered.

Smith emphasizes the importance of *caring* for dying patients when they are beyond the point where life can be preserved. Smith sees nurses and other health professionals as "healers and menders" of patients. He makes the significant point, however, that in caring for patients there are some dimensions of the patient's life that are beyond the professional's appropriate concern. These areas are more appropriate to the concern and attention of the family or the patient's "significant others" because these people are most intimately involved with the patient.[82] Concerns about decision making arise when nurses are caring for an individual who does not have family or significant others when particular problems that concern only the patient and family or significant others arise, and when it is inappropriate for health professionals to intervene. This becomes a particularly sensitive issue when the patient is unable to make these decisions; legal intervention may be necessary to secure a guardian or conservator.

Ramsey says that there is a duty never to abandon *care*. He says that in caring for the dying person one may eventually cease doing what was once called for and begin to do what is now required in the individual situation. This does not mean, according to Ramsey, that one is required to assist the dying process, but that one must assure the person that she or he is not alone and that others are aware of this dying and will be there during the dying process. Recall the needs and concerns of family members of dying persons. These caring values and practices are clearly demonstrated in the hospice movement. Ramsey also notes that we could formulate a moral rule that the *only* circumstance in which positive action might be taken to hasten a person's death is if there is the kind of prolonged dying where it is medically impossible to control the individual's pain or other distressing symptoms. The nurse, through close contact in caring for the patient and managing control of symptoms, may be the first to see that this situation has been reached by a particular patient. It becomes imperative for the nurse to communicate this to the patient's physician in response to an ethic of caring. The ethic and practice of allowing to die, recognized by most health professionals, still leaves the question as to whether physicians can take positive action to hasten death without weakening medicine's life-saving ethic.[83] It must also be noted that killing a patient is not an acceptable solution to poor symptom control.

A study of nurses' feelings about euthanasia was done at the University of Washington Hospital and Swedish Hospital Medical Center.[84] Findings indicated that nurses heard requests for positive or direct euthanasia from terminally ill patients and their families more frequently than did physicians. The underlying assumption was that nurses have more interaction with the patient and family than do physicians. More nurses were uncomfortable when physicians did not let patients irretrievably dying die than when the physician did follow this ethic. Nurses generally demonstrated more desire than physicians for social changes, such as legislation, to allow euthanasia. Eighty-five percent of the nurses surveyed stated that they would practice negative euthanasia with a signed statement of consent. This seems to demonstrate that nurses may hold the value that the patient has a right to maintain control and make decisions about the end of his life and his way of dying. More nurses than physicians supported the concept of using a committee or board for resolving difficult philosophical decisions about questions of euthanasia.

Nursing, as a profession, should articulate an ethic of care for the dying. Dyck's discussion of an ethic called benemortasia is of a happy or good death that is not necessarily painless or hastened by a physician's action. A moral distinction is made in this ethic between acts that *permit* death and acts that *cause* death.[85] According to this ethic, the compassion and freedom of the nurse are increased as the nurse cares for an irreversibly ill patient who has the freedom to refuse interventions that only prolong the dying process and to make choices such as how to live while dying. This ethic adheres to the commandment "thou shalt not kill" and stands in the deontological-ethical tradition. Nurses can help patients and families to look at hospice or hospice-like options for care, such as care at home when appropriate support is available. Nurses need to be particularly sensitive to families when home care is not a practicable choice. The author is aware of situations where home care has been imposed on families by well-meaning health professionals. The major focus should be on preserving the life and values of the human community, with mercy and compassion for the individual.

Nurses also work with patients who are, or are considered to be, suicidal. Suicide and assisting in suicide are generally considered to be unjustifiable acts of killing. Suicide, in one view, is considered to be the ultimate way of shutting out all other people from one's life and of saying that life is no longer worthwhile. This position negates the view that our lives are shaped by responses to others and their responses to us. This means we have responsibilities to others as members of groups and families. Suicide in any form negates this aspect of human community.[86]

In summary, the ethic of benemortasia maintains that[86]:

1. The individual's life is not solely at the disposal of that person, because he or she is part of a human community.
2. The individual has the freedom to make moral choices.
3. Every individual life has some worth.
4. The supreme value is goodness, in Western religious traditions referred to as God, to which the dying and those who care for the dying are responsible.

This involves the good of the individual and the community. No one human being or community can presume to know who should live or die. Dyck suggests that in carrying out this ethic, patients may need advocates other than physicians and nurses.[87] As there may be recognized conflict between the authority and autonomy of the health professionals and that of the patient, the patient needs someone outside of this conflict who represents his interests. Health professionals may adhere to the medical ethic that says one should do everything one can to preserve life. Death is seen as the failure of medical technology and knowledge. On the other hand, physicians sometimes determine when orders not to resuscitate are appropriate without consultation with the patient or family. In making patient care decisions, the nurse can and should act as an advocate for the competent patient's input and the family's input as appropriate.

The ethic of benemortasia, the points made by Smith, and the philosophy of the hospice movement provide starting points for discussion within and outside the profession by nurses confronted with a patient and family who want a respirator turned off or do not want heroic measures instituted. The Dying Person's Bill of Rights offers another framework for discussions and decision making about ethical issues that arise in the care of the dying person, whether an adult or a child.[88] The Dying Person's Bill of Rights includes such ideas as rights to treatment as a living human being until death, maintenance of a sense of hopefulness, expression of one's own feelings and emotions about approaching death, participation in decisions concerning one's care, freedom from pain, the right not to die alone, the right to have one's questions answered honestly without deception, the right to maintain one's individuality, and the right to be cared for by caring, sensitive, knowledgeable people. These "rights" parallel many of the needs identified by families of dying patients. The last right (to be cared for by caring, sensitive, knowledgeable people) implies that these people, including nurses, have deliberated on and continue to consider the ethical dimensions of questions posed by the availability of technologies that may or may not be used to maintain life.

To focus primarily on a patient-centered ethic, as we have done in this section, is not to ignore the hospital policy and public policy issues that arise in connection with society's priorities for health and illness and allocation of finite resources. Chapter 12 focuses on some ways that nursing is and can be actively involved in such areas as legislation, where death and dying create ethical dilemmas for health providers, consumers, legislators, and the human community at large.

Living wills for individuals also known as advance directives, hospital and nursing home guidelines for orders not to resuscitate, and court and legislative actions are all significant steps in seeking paths to resolving some of the ethical dilemmas that exist today concerning death and dying. Nurses should have opportunities to articulate and think through positions on these dilemmas that confront them as individuals and professionals. "Ethics rounds," courses in basic nursing education, and continuing education efforts in patient care ethics provide forums for doing this within the nursing community and with other health disciplines.

Nursing efforts in truly caring for the terminally ill and dying patient have made positive differences at the individual level of care and at the institutional policy level that are reflections of respect for persons. Concerns focus primarily on *how* to care for the dying patient rather than on whether one should treat or not treat.

REFERENCES

1. Gortner SR: Death with dignity: Ethical issues in the proposed legislation. *ANA Clinical Sessions, 1974*. New York: Appleton-Century-Crofts; 1975: p 169.
2. *Who Should Survive?*, film. Hartford, CT: Joseph P. Kennedy, Jr. Foundation Film Services; 1971.
3. Morison RS: Death: Process or event? In Steinfels P, Veatch RM (eds): *Death Inside Out: The Hastings Center Report*. New York: Harper & Row; 1974: p 68.
4. Report of the Ad Hoc Committee of the Harvard Medical School to Examine the Definition of Brain Death: A definition of irreversible coma. *JAMA* 205:85–88, 1968.
5. *Ibid.*, pp 86–87.
6. Kansas Statutes Annotated, C. 77-202, Definition of Death [L. 1970, c. 378.1:July 1]. Supplementary Pocket Part, p 45.
7. Capron AM: The Quinlan decision: Shifting the burden of decision making. *Hastings Cent Rep* 6:17, February 1976.
8. *Matter of Quinlan*, 70 NJ 10 (1976), 355 A2d 647 (NJ 1976).
9. Morison RS: *Death*, pp 65–69.
10. Kass LR: pp 73, 78.
11. Bok S: Lecture on severely defective newborns. Delivered in Ethics and Decision Making in Medicine, Harvard Medical School, January 19, 1977.
12. *Ibid.*
13. Duff RS, Campbell AGM: Moral and ethical dilemmas in the special-care nursery. *N Engl J Med* 289:890–894, 1973.
14. McCormick RA: To save or let die: The dilemma of modern medicine. *JAMA* 229:172–176, 1974.
15. Shaw A: Dilemmas of "informed consent" in children. *N Engl J Med* 289:885–890, 1973.
16. Ramsey P: *The Patient as Person*. New Haven: Yale University Press; 1970: pp 122–123.
17. Brody H: *Ethical Decisions in Medicine*. Boston: Little, Brown; 1976: p 72.
18. *Ibid.*
19. Ufema JK: Dare to care for the dying. *Am J Nurs* 76:89, 1976.

20. Simons SM: The obligation to live vs the option to die. *South Med J* 65:731, 1972.
21. *Kennedy Memorial Hospital v Heston*, 58 NJ 576. 279 A2d 670 (1972).
22. *Erickson v Dilgard*, 252 NY Supp. 2d 705 (1962).
23. Branson R, Casebeer K: The Quinlan decision: Obscuring the role of the physician. *Hastings Cent Rep* 6:9, February 1976.
24. Heifetz MS, Magel C: *The Right to Die*. New York: Putnam; 1975.
25. Fletcher GP: Legal aspects of the decision not to prolong life. *JAMA* 203:120, 1968.
26. Fletcher J: Ethics and euthanasia. *Am J Nurs* 73:670, 672, 1973.
27. Dyck AJ: Beneficent euthanasia and benemortasia: Alternative view of mercy. In Kohl M (ed): *Beneficent Euthanasia*. Buffalo, NY: Prometheus; 1975: p 120.
28. Mansson HH: Justifying the final solution. *Omega* 3:79–87, May 1972.
29. Fletcher J: Ethics and euthanasia, p 671.
30. Rawls J: *A Theory of Justice*. Cambridge, MA: Harvard University Press; 1971: pp 131–135.
31. Dyck AJ: Beneficent euthanasia, pp 124–125.
32. Weber LJ: Ethics and euthanasia: Another view. *Am J Nurs* 73:1228–1230, 1973.
33. Kamisar Y: From euthanasia legislation: Some nonreligious objections. In Gorovitz S, et al (eds): *Moral Problems in Medicine*. Englewood Cliffs, NJ: Prentice-Hall; 1976: p 402.
34. Brody H: *Ethical Decisions*, p 195.
35. Heifetz MD, Magel C: *Right to Die*, pp 111–112.
36. Weber LF: Ethics and euthanasia, p 1231.
37. White RB: Case studies in bioethics: A demand to die. *Hastings Cent Rep* June 1975.
38. Reich W: The physician's "duty" to preserve life. *Hastings Cent Rep* 5:15, April 1975.
39. Weber LJ: Ethics and euthanasia, pp 1229–1231.
40. Pontoppidan H: Optimum care for hopelessly ill patients. *N Engl J Med*, 295:362–364, 1976.
41. Rabkin MT, Gillerman G, Rice NR: Orders not to resuscitate. *N Engl J Med* 295:364–366, 1976.
42. *A Living Will*. New York: Concern for Dying.
43. Bok S: Personal directions for care at the end of life. *N Engl J Med* 295:368–369, 1976.
44. Garland M: The right to die in California: Politics, legislation, and natural death. *Hastings Cent Rep* October 1976.
45. Duff RS, Campbell AGM: Moral and ethical dilemmas, pp 890–894.
46. Shaw A: Dilemmas of "informed consent," p 885–890.
47. Kluge FHW: *The Practice of Death*. New Haven: Yale University Press; 1975: pp 182–209.
48. Zachary RB: Ethical and social aspects of treatment of spina bifida. In Gorovitz S, et al (eds): *Moral Problems in Medicine*. Englewood Cliffs, NJ: Prentice-Hall; 1976: pp 343–352.
49. Freeman JM: Is there a right to die quickly? In Gorovitz S, et al (eds): *Moral Problems in Medicine*. Englewood Cliffs, NJ: Prentice-Hall; 1976: pp 354–356.

50. Engelhardt T, Jr: Aiding the death of young children. In Kohl M (ed): *Beneficent Euthanasia*. Buffalo, NY, Prometheus; 1975: pp 180–192.
51. Robertson JA: Dilemma in Danville. *Hastings Cent Rep* 11:8, October 1981.
52. Heifetz MD, Magel C: *Right to Die*, p 71.
53. Heifetz MD, Magel C: *Ibid.*, p 79.
54. Kant I: Duties towards the body in regard to life. In Gorovitz S, et al (eds): *Moral Problems in Medicine*. Englewood Cliffs, NJ: Prentice-Hall; 1976: pp 376–377.
55. Williams G: From the right to commit suicide. In Gorovitz S, et al (eds): *Moral Problems in Medicine*. Englewood Cliffs, NJ: Prentice-Hall; 1976: p 388.
56. Murphy GE: Suicide and the right to die. In Gorovitz S, et al (eds): *Moral Problems in Medicine*. Englewood Cliffs, NJ: Prentice-Hall; 1976: p 387–388.
57. Rockwell DA, O'Brien W: Physicians' knowledge and attitudes about suicide. *JAMA* 225:1347–1349, 1973.
58. Heifetz MD, Magel C: *Right to Die*, pp 81, 96.
59. Berger P, Hamburg B, Hamburg D: Mental health: Progress and problems. *Daedalus* Winter 1977, p 270.
60. Murphy GE: Suicide and the right to die, pp 387–388.
61. Hook S: The ethics of suicide. In Kohl M (ed): *Beneficent Euthanasia*. Buffalo, NY: Prometheus; 1975: pp 60–63.
62. *Ibid.*, pp 66–67.
63. Quint JC: *The Nurse and the Dying Patient*. New York: Macmillan; 1967.
64. Quint JC: The threat of death: Some consequences for patients and nurses. *Nurs Forum* 8:287–300, 1969.
65. Strauss AL, Glasser BG: *Anguish: A Case History of a Dying Trajectory*. Mill Valley, CA: Sociology Press; 1970.
66. Yeaworth RC, Kapp FT, Winget C: Attitudes of nursing students toward the dying patient. *Nurs Res* 23:20–24, 1974.
67. Lester D, Getty C, Kneisl CR: Attitudes of nursing students and nursing faculty toward death. *Nurs Res* 23:50–59, 1974.
68. Griffin JJ: Family decision: A crucial factor in terminating life. *Am J Nurs* 75:794–796, 1975.
69. Kuhn MF: Death and dying: The right to live—the right to die. *ANA Clinical Session 1974*. New York: Appleton-Century-Crofts; 1975: pp 184–189.
70. Schorr TM: Editorial: The right to die. *Am J Nurs* 76:53, 1976.
71. Caughil RE (ed): *The Dying Patient: A Supportive Approach*. Boston: Little, Brown; 1976.
72. Hershey N: On the question of prolonging life. *Am J Nurs* 71:521–522, 1971.
73. Rabkin MT, Gillerman G, Rice NR: Orders not to resuscitate, pp 365–366.
74. Assell RA: If you were dying. In Caughill RE (ed): *The Dying Patient: A Supportive Approach*. Boston: Little, Brown; 1976: pp 47–71.
75. Gortner GR: Growing up to dying: The child, the parents, and the nurse. In Caughil RE (ed): *The Dying Patient: A Support Approach*. Boston: Little Brown; 1976: pp 159–189.
76. Hampe S: Needs of the grieving spouse in a hospital setting. *Nurs Res* 24:116–117, 1975.
77. Michaels DR: Too much in need of support to give any? *Nurs Res* 21:286, 1972.

78. Strank RA: Caring for the chronic sick and dying: A study of attitudes. *Nurs Times* 68:116–169, 1972.
79. Gortner SR: Growing up, p 175.
80. Smith DH: Some ethical considerations in caring for the dying. ANA Clinical Sessions, 1974. New York: Appleton-Century-Crofts; 1975: pp 177–178, 181.
81. Ramsey P: *Patient as Person*, pp 116–117.
82. Smith DH: Some ethical considerations, pp 180–181.
83. Ramsey P: *Patient as Person*, pp 153, 164.
84. Brown NK, Donovan JT, Bulger RJ, et al: How do nurses feel about euthanasia and abortion? *Am J Nurs* 71:1415–1416, 1971.
85. Dyck AJ: An alternative to the ethics of euthanasia. In Williams RH (ed): *To Live and to Die: When, Why, and How.* New York: Springer; 1974: pp 102–104.
86. *Ibid.*, pp 104, 106, 111.
87. *Ibid.*, pp 109, 111.
88. Barbus AJ: The dying person's bill of rights. *Am J Nurs* 75:99, 1975.

CHAPTER 10

Behavior Control

The long history of social evolution has engaged the human species in an endless struggle to understand, predict, influence, and control human behavior. The notion of the common good has been invoked in most instances for coercing an individual to conform to social mores. Historically, the tyranny of the majority has had limited results, especially in private life, since the machinery of repression has had no efficient ways to cope with the deviance and nonconformity engaged in within the confines of an individual's own home and in private relationships. Laws developed to deal with this area of life to a large extent functioned more as expressions of public morality than as incursions on private liberty. However, recently developed control methods make it possible now to exact conformity with greater reliability and less potential for resistance than has been the case in the past. Increasingly we have the technology to effectively engineer consent, which can thereby eliminate personal license and still leave individuals with the feeling that they are free. This situation may appeal as a therapeutic tool to those who work with the "hard-core" criminal or the severely mentally ill; however, such developments in behavior control, with widespread use, can also serve to unhinge the conventional political morality essential to modern democracy. The basic ethical problem of behavior control arises in the dilemma of how to maintain personal liberty in situations where suppression of liberty can be rationalized not only by the needs of the common welfare but also by the individual's happiness.

The potential success of behavior control techniques to change people—prison inmates, mental patients, and the entire gamut of people seeking psychiatric help with the goal of self-fulfillment and self-realization—has become the source of controversy within the larger debate as to society's proper response to deviant behavior. The concept of unintended consequences, which maintains that reforms and innovations often carry with them effects of a social nature contrary to the stated purpose of the intended goals, becomes a central concern in developing techniques to control behavior.[1] For example, according to sociologists and social historians, the original intent in establishing asylums for the mentally ill, which was to provide a protective setting with treatment and humane conditions, also had the unintentional consequence of turning them into warehouses for the mentally ill where loss of individuality, depersonalization, and dehumanization resulted.[2-4] The concerns surrounding behavior control and the unintended consequences can be understood in the context of the three social dilemmas that prisons and mental hospitals share: (1) How does the institutional social structure affect attempts at treatment and rehabilitation? (2) How can these institutions meet both the demands of society and the needs of the individuals they serve? (3) What kind of control should be exercised over the development and application of behavior control techniques? Although the criminal justice system and the mental health system both use forms of behavior control, for the most part this chapter will focus on the latter.

During the 1950s and 1960s we came to recognize that prisons and mental hospitals fall far short of meeting the goals set for them by society. Critics, both in and out of the mental health field, traced this failure to a number of variables, including the basic factor that the social structure of these institutions not only did not always support their stated goals but at times tended to undermine their purpose.[5-8] The recognition of these problems led to three changes that affected the "total institution" nature of the mental hospital. In an attempt to alter the social structure of mental hospitals, Jones developed the therapeutic community concept in the United Kingdom, which became a major reform movement during the 1950s and 1960s.[9-10] The second change, the community mental health movement, arose from an awareness of the negative aspects of maintaining a patient in a total institution over a long period of time. This change resulted in a shift away from almost total reliance on public institutions with their involuntary incarceration and treatment to a more voluntaristic and pluralistic system. The third change, which made the first two possible, has been the development of behavior control technology, all of which has become more sophisticated, more effective, and more efficient. This technology includes psychotropic drugs, electroshock therapy, psychosurgery, behavior modification, and other psychological techniques. This fundamental change, developments in technology, has raised basic legal and ethical questions regarding the rights of patients and the role of staff members in a situation where some view psychiatric personnel as double agents—that is, as regulatory agents for the state and as therapeutic agents for the patient. This can, and does, create a conflict-of-interest problem.[11,12]

Before proceeding to a more detailed discussion of specific forms of behavior control, it will be helpful to define the term itself and to consider the fundamental problems of deviancy and coercion. London defined behavior control as getting people to do someone else's bidding, as has been depicted in several fictional and nonfiction accounts.[13-18] In the broadest sense, behavior control can be understood as a special form of behavioral change. For example, in a psychiatric setting, treatment offered to or imposed on a patient may to a large extent be designed to satisfy the wishes of others. Behavioral change that satisfies others—the community or society, for example—may or may not satisfy the patient's wishes to change. The use of behavior control with the mentally ill has been questioned on the grounds that such treatment deprives patients of the fundamental right to choose their course of action. As behavior control technology develops and becomes more available, and as the psychiatric categories seem to expand to include more attitudes and behaviors defined as deviant, numerous ethical questions arise. Preventive psychiatry continues to define more and more problems of human behavior as falling within its jurisdiction, yet the critics maintain that its practitioners are unable to cope with its present scope. This inability to deliver the goods, so to speak, may be considered as both an ethical problem and a safeguard against unchecked power. With recent research probing the biological base of major mental illnesses, some of the ethical questions for the future will be different from those that are central in behavior control today.

DEVIANCY AND MENTAL ILLNESS

Every society has its rules and social norms. It is generally expected in a given society that a majority of the people will conform to these rules and norms most of the time. In addition, every society has its nonconformists, who may be artists with their bohemian life-style, which most communities within society will tolerate without attempting to control as long as such a life-style does not deviate too much from the established norm. The nonconformists usually considered as deviants and social problems in our society do not constitute a homogeneous group, and the characteristics that bring them societal attention do not lend themselves to easy classification. Generally speaking, the most obvious groups considered deviant in our own society fall into the following nonexclusive categories: medical (the mentally ill); intellectual (the mentally retarded); chronological (the senile); social (the alcoholic); economic (other drug abusers); sexual (the homosexual); or doctrinal nonconformity (the sociopolitical radical). These groups share two things in common. First, their behavior is proscribed or controlled by law, and second, society increasingly seeks them out for "treatment" instead of "punishment."[19] It is of importance to note that sexual deviants who are homosexuals have been eliminated from this category by a vote of psychiatrists. Such an action demonstrates how social norms change and influence the definition of what is deviant. It also shows the fluidity of the boundaries between normal and abnormal behavior. Basically, social groups create deviance when they make rules whose infraction constitutes deviance and when they apply those rules to particular individuals and label them as outsiders. It follows, then, that deviance is not a quality of the act the person commits, but rather a consequence of the application by others of rules and sanctions to a so-called offender. The deviant person is one to whom that label has successfully been applied and deviant behavior is behavior that people so labeled engage in, according to a classic study on this topic.[20]

Those persons whom we call mentally ill tend to be at variance with the mores and conventions of society. The fact that this condition usually has behavioral rather than physiological symptoms alone casts those so labeled into the role of the social deviant. Mental illness is not easy to define or to determine, and this situation becomes compounded by the fact that different societies may have different tolerance levels for the sort of deviation that becomes labeled as mental illness.

The concept *dangerousness* has been the paramount consideration in the legal commitment procedure within our mental health system. That means that for the mentally ill deviant, the only legitimate justification for civil commitment was thought to be a provable likelihood of dangerous acts toward the self or toward others. However, the mental health field does not possess the tools to determine, with any degree of precision, those who will be dangerous. Dangerousness, like any number of other things, including beauty, is, to some extent, in the eye of the beholder. Although the general public has tended to associate dangerousness with mental illness, the American Psychiatric Association has indicated that about 10% of the hospitalized mentally ill can be considered dangerous.[21] However, according to other sources, this figure of 10% may be grossly inflated. The base rate of violent behavior (except for suicide) by those labeled mentally ill is no different than for the general population.

Numerous experts have pointed to the inadequacy of the criteria for predicting who will commit a dangerous act.[22-25] Some critiques of the predictive techniques emphasize that violent behavior is not only a function of personality but also a function of social context. This provides one explanation as to why the traditional psychiatric approach, which emphasizes personality, would have limited predictive value.[26,27] The above comments are not intended to imply that no traditional psychiatric clues are valid, only that such validity has yet to be established. The difficulty involved in predicting dangerousness increases when the patient has never actually performed an assaultive act. This problem obviously becomes particularly relevant to involuntary hospitalization situations. Some believe that mental health professionals, since they have no reliable criteria, tend to overpredict dangerousness. In such instances, so the argument goes, these professionals have stereotyped ideas of the personality attributes of dangerous individuals that have no valid relationship to the occurrence of dangerous acts. Rather, they commit themselves to these stereotypes because of theoretical constructs that cause them to attend selectively to certain data. In addition to the problems of identification and prediction of dangerous behavior, some, including the National Council on Crime and Delinquency, maintain that neither mental hospitals nor prisons are now capable of treating persons labeled as dangerous. It must be seen as a bizarre system of criminal justice that confines mostly those who cannot be identified as dangerous, and equally bizarre a mental health system that commits mostly those who cannot be treated.

A study conducted by a nurse explored the notion that the concept of dangerousness is a social construction. The study focus was an examination of how nursing personnel on locked inpatient psychiatric units define patients as dangerous to others.[28]

COERCION AND FREEDOM

The following comments come from an essay by William Gaylin, a psychoanalyst who has been for many years the president of the Hastings Center, one of the two think tanks in bioethics in the United States. He points out that in the United States freedom constitutes a dominant value; however, the structure of organized society depends on defined limits of freedom. The legal system supplies the definitions of permissible behavior and also establishes the coercion force that society may use to ensure compliance. Therefore, coercion may not necessarily always be an evil. The basis of civilization depends to a great extent on the right of the state to coerce its citizens. These statements lead to the realization that we must weigh society's right to coerce against the individual's right to freedom. Furthermore, one needs to think through what constitutes a coerced, as distinguished from a free, act. Freedom, a principle to which psychiatry aspires rather than a concept that it often employs, has not been incorporated to any extent into a theory of behavior, since psychiatry has difficulty fitting freedom with theory that tends toward a deterministic view. With a frame of reference that defines a person as less than rational and motivated more by appeals to emotions than by appeals to reason, psychiatry, and especially psychoanalysis, is far more comfortable with the concept of coercion.[29]

Since those things that people experience are true determinants of behavior, the perception of danger becomes the crucial issue in coercion. To understand coercion one must understand that which threatens man. The problem is not so much the coercion involved in physical force and threatening survival itself, but threats to survival equivalents, such as threat of isolation, loss of love, social humiliation, and so on.

As stated earlier, the social order relies to some extent on the right to coercion. Along with the legal dimensions of coercion, society has given a moral privilege to coercion when such action is done in the individual's best interest. For example, certain parental behavior coerces children, but society permits this because of the assumption that parents have the child's best interest at heart. Also, in the field of health, coercion has a traditional respectability and legal sanction, and psychiatry, as a branch of medicine, has engaged in coercion. Indeed, one might correctly say that, in the recent past, the abrogation of the legal rights of the mentally ill, the denial of due process, and the confinement beyond the limits the law tolerates for criminals represent a gross example of coercion.

Behavior control represents a broad spectrum of activities, including psychiatric therapy, political propaganda, commercial advertising, religious and moral education, and rehabilitation of deviant persons. The major categories of behavior control in the mental health field that will be discussed in this chapter are psychotherapy, psychosurgery, and psychopharmacology. Practitioners in the field readily accept the fact that patients should be protected from outright coercion, and this belief has been formalized in statutes and regulations. The idea that the patient should also be protected from more subtle pressures is not only more difficult for many mental health professionals to accept, but makes the problems of such regulation more difficult as well.

PSYCHOTHERAPY

Psychotherapy has gone through three developmental stages during the 20th century. Each of these stages has been in response to the psychosocial motif dominating the society at that time. Stage one came into being with the development of psychoanalysis. This occurred around the beginning of this century, when Freud and Breuer first published their works and formed the Psychoanalytic Society in 1902. Psychoanalysis treated by uncovering and exposing unconscious material that had been repressed. The patients, mostly middle class women, lived in the Victorian era of Vienna, known for its standards of proper behavior and repression of sexuality. Psychoanalysis came into being in this era to deal with its major psychosocial motif. One problem identified with all psychotherapeutic approaches requiring long-term therapy has been the lack of evidence to prove its effectiveness for patients. Traditional psychodynamic therapies have not produced empiric validation of the treatment efficacy. Two problems arise with attempts to research this area. The first problem is defining what is to be measured, which rests on the larger problem of the definition of normal or healthy. The second problem concerns methodology, or ways of evaluating possible long-range effects of psychotherapy on both individuals and society as a whole. Psychotherapy of any type can occur between a middle class patient and therapist who share more or less similar attitudes and values, and this process may be a voluntary activity chosen by the patient. However, it can also occur as an involuntary activity when the patient, who may or may not share values and attitudes with the therapist, becomes legally committed. Therapy has been viewed as a political act in either case, in that the therapist can encourage patients to either adjust to or rebel against their environment. However, the potential for using psychotherapy as a coercive tool of social control increases in the situation of involuntary commitment. Psychotherapy can be based on the social and economic biases of the therapist rather than the patient's behavior, and as such can become a coercive tool operating mainly on those very groups that are least able to change the social context in which their problems arise.

Stage two occurred during the 1950s and 1960s with the development of psychotherapy based on principles of conditioning. The generalized term, behavior modification, became the generic name for those methods emphasizing a behavioristic orientation. Another activist treatment, crisis intervention, led to the establishment of crisis intervention centers where clients could come in or telephone at any time in an attempt to deal with their problems. These two approaches shared several things: direct attack on the symptoms presented, without going into the underlying cause; short duration of therapy; and the possibility of a more technological basis for therapy than had been available in previous therapeutic approaches. Stage two represents a shift away from treating causes to an era of treatment geared toward symptom relief.

Stage three grew out of the affluence and leisure that the large middle class had achieved in the late 1960s and the early 1970s, when society passed from the age of anxiety to the age of ennui. The overriding preoccupation for many became the achievement of value and meaning in life. Psychotherapy shifted away from a focus on the relief of discomfort and pain to meeting the demands of the populace who sought a richer life with deeper experiences and relationships. At present, the developments from all three stages continue to function to meet the different needs of a vast number of individuals with a great variety of reasons for seeking help or having it imposed on them. As indicated for Stage one, the developments in Stages two and three, separately or in combination, can also serve as coercive tools of social control.

In addition to these stages, we also have present problems, clinical, social, and ethical. Among these are the homeless mentally ill and the large numbers of the young chronically mentally ill who often have dual diagnoses as a result of their mental illness and drug taking. These populations represent a failure in the social movement of deinstitutiona- lization. The goal was to empty the mental hospitals and have the mentally ill enter into society, with both ethical and economic consider- ations being under debate.

Other problems have arisen more recently and our society has de- clared war on drugs. The fact that great numbers of people are addicted to drugs of all types and that newborn babies begin their lives addicted has grave potential consequences for society and certainly raises numer- ous ethical issues. For example, should drugs be legalized? Should abusers who are apprehended by the police be forced to enter treatment programs, and who will pay for such programs? Should bus drivers, truck drivers, and others whose jobs may do harm to others if per- formed under the influence of drugs, undergo drug testing in order to retain those jobs? Should pregnant women who are on drugs either have an abortion or be placed in a treatment program? What obligations does society have to these babies? These problems do not easily fall into a stage, perhaps because we are too close to them and do not have the benefit of a longer view. However, taken together they demonstrate the dynamic interaction among the concepts of democracy, social definitions and issues, behavior control questions, and ethical dilemmas.

Behavior control, as a potential ethical dilemma, varies with the different methods of treatment used. Psychotherapy has been widely accepted and practiced as the major means therapists have to deal with psychological disorders. It has been less recognized or discussed as a means of controlling people. Long-term insight therapy can be utilized systematically to influence attitudes and values, if not overt behavior, toward conventional norms of conduct. One could however, make the argument, that because this therapy method is slow, technologically benign, and limited to a relatively small target population, the risks incurred, as far as behavior control goes, are few. As behavior changes occur, the patient develops an accompanying increase in his awareness, enabling him to monitor his own behavior changes to some extent. Furthermore, to a large degree, clients participating in insight therapy remain outside the large mental hospitals, so that the factors of institu- tional social structure do not affect the attempt at treatment and rehabil- itation.

Stage two, with its principles of conditioning, deserves more atten- tion since such treatment techniques have been rigorously criticized as being repressive and dehumanizing.[30] Our fascination with technology leads us to overrate the promise as well as the threat of these new techniques. Such techniques received attention in the controversial film of Anthony Burgess' novel, Clockwork Orange.[31] Generally speaking, the type of behavior control referred to as behavior therapy or behavior modification is one in which the therapist manipulates the environment and the consequences of a person's behavior in order to change that behavior, otherwise called operant conditioning. The therapist reinforces desired behavior whereas the behavior not wanted receives an adverse response or, at a minimum, receives no reward. A classic report of Ivar Lovaas's work with autistic children who had not been reached by normal methods of love, compassion, and punishment provides us with an example of behavior modification. The therapist placed barefoot autistic children in a room with a metal grid in the floor. The children periodically received an electric shock that they could avoid only by throwing themselves into the arms of an adult. After a time, these children began to seek out adults on their own without the shock. Another example involved a young boy who had been strapped to his bed for more than 7 years. When he was not strapped to the bed, he would take bites out of his shoulder. After three severe electrical jolts with a cattle prod, he stopped the biting behavior. Upon return to his usual ward, however, he reverted to his previous behavior. The physician visited the ward and discovered that as soon as the boy tried to bite himself, the nurse would immediately run up and lovingly hug him, thereby rewarding his abnormal biting behavior. Such behavior modification techniques as described here may seem cruel, and indeed may be. Yet, in the second example, the case of misapplied love maintained a situation that also could be viewed as cruel.[32]

Success using this type of therapy has been rather limited because of the major difficulty in retaining changed behavior over time. However, the success obtained in the treatment of chronic patients has been accomplished with behavioral techniques. The larger question that arises has to do with the possible gains as against the possible losses. Considerable evidence that people's behavior can be programmed fairly easily now exists. One basic premise underlying much current research seems to be that man is after all an animal, and many features of his learning and behavior share similarities with those found in a large number of animals. The argument goes that it should be possible to train a human by the same methods that have been so well developed for animals—rats, dogs, and pigeons, for example. In general, behavior therapy and behavior modification methods have been shown to be somewhat superior to other forms of therapy; however, difficult disorders do not produce very positive results, and no evidence shows that the effects persist over time. These comments must be considered with the realization that most, if not all, psychotherapeutic techniques have limitations, so alternatives may or may not exist. Traditional methods of treating hospitalized psychiatric patients, including individual therapy, group therapy, work therapy, and drug therapy, do not differentially affect the discharge patients' community functioning as measured by recidivism and posthospital employment. But in recent years, with the development of community mental health programs, many patients receive treatment outside hospitals. However, this development has not solved the baffling problems of major mental illness. These programs' major techniques, individual and group therapy, have had limited effectiveness, at best, and they either do not reach or are inimical to major segments of the population requiring help. In short, any criticism of behavior therapy must take into account the ethical dilemmas involved but must also allow for the state of the science and art of psychiatry. This entire situation has been exacerbated by the fact that in formulating new rules of mental health, the professionals have created new classes of mentally ill individuals to the extent that we may possibly today have an exaggeration of the concept of mental illness.

Behavior modification has been greatly influenced by Skinnerian behaviorism with its emphasis on environmental control and shaping of behavior.[33,34] The antibehaviorism viewpoint, developed early as a reaction to behavior modification and expressed in the writings of Carl Rogers and others, including Jourard, contends that while the so-called behavioristic approach to psychiatry acknowledges an individual's susceptibility to manipulation by another, it also ignores the possible deleterious impact of this manipulation on the whole person and, in addition, on the manipulator himself.[35,36] They believe that the essential factor in the psychotherapeutic encounter is an honest, loving, spontaneous relationship between the therapist and patient.[37-39] On the other hand, a behavioristic point of view could make the argument that apparent spontaneity of the therapist's part can well be the most effective means of manipulating the patient's behavior. The therapist has been programmed by his training into a fairly effective behavior control machine of sorts, and most likely this machine is most effective when it appears least like a machine. To summarize this point, a science of psychology of psychiatry seeks to determine the lawful relationships in behavior, while the science of behavior control rests on the assumption that these relationships are to be used to deliberately influence, control, or change behavior. This orientation implies a controller who has an ethical and value system. However, the reciprocity of the relationship between the controller and the controlled, an important facet of behavior control, often goes overlooked.

PSYCHOSURGERY

While psychosurgery, or surgery to alter behavior, has been a topic of discussion in scientific literature, congressional reports, legal documents, and lay publications, it has not received much attention recently, perhaps because of a greater reliance on drugs for the mentally ill. Nevertheless, it is important to examine this topic for a more historical view to understand the ethical issues involved. The general term *psychosurgery* refers to a number of surgical procedures, such as cingulotomy, amygdalatomy, thalamotomy, lobotomy, and lobectomy. In 1970, a neurosurgeon and a psychiatrist wrote a book entitled *Violence and the Brain* that detailed the application of neurosurgery techniques to the problems of violent behavior.[40] The response to this book vividly underscored the growing concern with the social role of such experts who have within their power, along with the geneticist, the possibility of turning the classic philosophical question, "What is man?" to a very different question, "What kind of man are we going to construct?" In reaction to the response, Vernon Mark, the neurosurgeon, and philosopher Robert Neville, offered some reflections on the social issues involved in psychosurgery, making the point that most criticisms either impute to this type of surgery more capability than it can deliver or assume that such surgery would be appropriate to use for control in those instances when no surgeon would agree to such a use.[41] Psychosurgery, like any other technology, can be misused; nevertheless, the basic problem stems from the dichotomy in fundamental approaches to behavior.

Many social scientists and others in the mental health field view certain behavioral abnormalities, such as aggressive, assaultive behavior or intractable depression, as resulting from unusual or abnormal environmental stress and feel that brain function or dysfunction does not play a part in abnormal behavior. Obviously, no human behavior, normal or abnormal, can be the consequence of the brain alone without the environment and equally obviously, no behavior, whatever its environmental determinants, occurs without the brain freighting its mechanical impulses with emotion and culture. A statement that recognizes the brain's involvement in behavior does not lead to the conclusion, as some critics think, that all behavior should be controlled through the brain.

Mark and Neville continue by developing three alternative defenses of psychosurgical procedures, which illustrate their theses regarding the appropriateness of this type of behavior control.[41] Importantly, they reject the first two alternatives. Alternative one states that medical means should be undertaken to improve any behavior, normal or abnormal, whenever possible. This position has the advantage of avoiding the difficult task of defining normality and the disadvantage of making medicine the authority on improvement, of what constitutes the good life and the proper means of achieving it. Alternative two states that any undesirable, abnormal behavior should be treated by whatever medical means available, including psychosurgery, if it can be shown to be the most efficient method with the least risk. Two problems arise with this position. First, psychiatric neurosurgery, despite great technical advances, is still experimental and irreversible. The second problem, that a person will be set up for psychosurgery simply because someone else does not desire his behavior, received a dramatic treatment in the book and film, *One Flew Over the Cuckoo's Nest*.[42] Alternative three, accepted by Mark and Neville, states that drastic procedures such as psychosurgery should be used only when behavior is abnormal and "bad" primarily because of a brain abnormality. Then any abnormal behavior not associated with brain disease will be dealt with by political and social means, not medical ones.

The point must be made before leaving this topic that environmental cues controlled many in the German population to the extent that they played at least a passive part in one of the worst scenes of carnage ever enacted on the human stage. Some would argue that the human personality and brain, programmed specifically for environmental inputs and controls, receives its most outstanding threat for behavior control from that which already exists and not from psychosurgery or drugs.

PSYCHOPHARMACOLOGY

At this point, every informed person in the United States must know about both the pharmacological developments potentially enabling us to control human emotions and mental functioning and the extent of drug use in this country. At one time, we commonly thought of psychotropic drugs as for use with patients diagnosed as psychotic or depressed. More recently it has been found that relatively normal people increasingly use these agents to cope with the stresses encountered in daily life. Statistics indicate that the production and distribution of psychotropic drugs have become a major component of the drug industry. The 1967 estimates of 180 million prescriptions for these drugs at a cost of 700 million dollars give us some idea of the magnitude of the situation. Data from one study conducted in California indicate that approximately 17 percent of adults reported frequent use of psychotropic drugs, with the figure being twice as high for females as for men and with the heaviest use occurring in the 40- to 59-year-old age group.[43] Over two decades have passed since those figures were reported. Since that time the concern over the quantity of prescription drugs has been replaced by the crisis of and national war on illegal drugs. The most dramatic event in the war on these drugs was the United States invasion of Panama in December 1989. This drug subculture has grown to such an extent that it has become a major social, economic, and mental health problem for the country.

Psychopharmacology emerged as a separate branch within pharmacology after World War II, with the discovery of LSD (lysergic diethylamide) in 1943 and chlorpromazine in 1952. During the next few years, and with great rapidity, dozens of new compounds became available. Psychotropic drugs have been divided into three categories, depending on the purpose for which they are used: (1) drugs used as therapeutic agents for the treatment of psychiatric disorders; (2) drugs used for nontherapeutic purposes, such as recreation or personal enjoyment; and (3) drugs used to enhance performance and capabilities. In each category ethical issues arise, including that of coercion, which can be a special problem in category one. Because of the decentralized character of drug taking, the necessity for repeated doses, and the fact that pills are often self-administered, the problem of behavior control through drugs is less of an issue than getting people not to take these drugs. Of all the techniques that modern technology has developed and that can be used for controlling behavior, drugs are certainly among the most widely disseminated and readily available. In a drug culture, where many people think a visit to the doctor's office or clinic has been a waste of time unless they come away with some pills and where the medical professional usually reinforces this attitude, the possibility of drug abuse of all kinds, including behavior control, can pose the single most difficult problem because of availability, accessibility, and the general cultural attitude.

At the same time that concern over taking drugs has increased, there is more discussion about the rights of the mentally ill to refuse medication and state laws to ensure those rights.[44,45]

ETHICAL DILEMMAS

The right to receive treatment and the right to refuse treatment in general, and the right to consent to or decline behavior modification techniques in particular, raise a conflict-of-interest question. Does the therapist satisfy his own interests or those of the patients or, most likely, some combination of the two? In some situations, the therapist serves a third party, and this can be a problem, especially when he is an employee of an institution whose interests do not necessarily coincide with the interests of the patient. Third parties often apply subtle and sometimes not so subtle pressures that therapists may not be fully aware of or understand. Conflict of interest represents one facet of the wider problem of what values, especially what conflicting values, are served by the mental health field. One major obstacle to a greater awareness of these value conflicts comes from the fact that mental health professionals have a marked tendency to assume that they function in a value-free frame of reference. Keenly aware of the patient's conflicts, they may be less inclined to see the conflicts of their own social role. The fact remains that regardless of theoretical orientation, these professionals are often a party to such conflict.

The larger ethical question involved in behavior control of any type turns on the problem of personal integrity. The essential question then is, does the individual have an inviolable, indefeasible, absolute right to be himself, whatever or whoever he is, the product of whatever heredity and environment is his lot, even if he is deviant or dangerous to himself or others? A whole host of questions for consideration in discussing behavior control include: If the individual is dangerous to himself, does society have the right to intervene to stop him from hurting or destroying himself? Does society have the right or obligation to protect its members from themselves or from others? On what moral ground can the limit be determined where individual rights become outweighed by societal rights? Who will decide who is dangerous and on the basis of what knowledge? How is normalcy to be defined for therapy? If a social deviant receives psychiatric treatment, should the aim of that treatment be adjustment or adaptation? Are there ethical grounds for rejecting some or all of the more potent behavior control techniques, even if they prove to be quite effective? When are possible risks from such procedures justified? How is consent obtained and from whom? Is experimentation justified outside of the context of a reasonable belief that the procedure will be therapeutic for the individual? If therapists increasingly use these techniques, should there be some type of regulation device over and beyond informed consent? One way to answer the last question is that any treatment recommendation for civilly committed disturbed patients who have not consented that involves brain surgery, electric shock therapy, prolonged use of drugs, or behavior therapy should be reviewed and approved by a monitoring agency. Who will be on this monitoring agency and who will select the members? Other questions are: Should such treatment as long-term use of psychotropic drugs or psychosurgery be considered for children? If so, which children will be eligible for this treatment and who will decide on what grounds? Is it ethical to deny such treatment to adults or children if all other treatment approaches have failed? Should such a technique as brain surgery be used as a means to control violent behavior, even if such behavior is of unknown cause? How does any one of these behavior control techniques determine the relationship between the patient and his doctor, nurse, or family? How does the technology affect the distribution of monetary and other resources for medical care? Who pays for such treatment? What are the possible potential implications of behavior control?

Essentially, the ethical questions boil down to: What kind of behavior should be controlled? Whose behavior is controlled? Who controls? Who decides who controls? How does behavior control affect dignity and freedom? What are the costs of gaining self-control? What social interests justify social control? What instruments of control are warranted to serve the interest of society? All of these questions evolve from several ethical dilemmas involved in behavior control. The dilemma of maintaining personal integrity versus society's obligation to protect its members remains perhaps the most central dilemma. The dilemma of immunity versus forfeiture of rights raises the question of what rights to privacy and inviolability of body and mind a person should lose once he has been diagnosed as mentally ill, especially if he is committed to an institution. The dilemma of procedural rights is concerned with what rights a patient has to the procedural protection from the suspension, waiver, or forfeiture of these basic rights. The dilemma of rights and goods concerns the possible conflict between the person's right to be different and his potential desire to be free from any misery that his deviance causes. The dilemma of informed voluntary consent raises the problems of mental status and legal status as inhibitions to obtaining informed consent. The dilemma of paternalism and authoritarianism raises the questions that John Stuart Mill addressed: What are the limits on the use of coercion, on the kinds of coercion, and on the actions coercively prevented or elicited that one person may use on another in the name of the latter's own good? The fact that those using the techniques of intervention may be doing so with therapeutic intent does not alter either the paternalistic or the authoritarian character of such use under certain circumstances. The dilemma of deceptive labeling concerns the issue of when enforced treatment, especially that involving irreversible effects, becomes primitive control under a false therapeutic label.

In 1971 Kittrie developed a Therapeutic Bill of Rights because he believed that the philosophical origins of therapeutic programs combined humanism, paternalism, and utilitarian determinism in promoting the public's interest in social defense. This document is fundamental to the ethical issues involved in behavior control today. The general principles of the Therapeutic Bill of Rights are[46]:

1. No person shall be compelled to undergo treatment except for the defense of society.
2. Man's innate right to remain free of excessive forms of human modification shall be inviolable.
3. No social sanctions may be invoked unless the person subjected to treatment has demonstrated a clear and present danger through truly harmful behavior which is immediately forthcoming or has already occurred.
4. No person shall be subjected to involuntary incarceration or treatment on the basis of a finding of a general condition of status alone. Nor shall the mere conviction for a crime or a finding of not guilty by reason of insanity suffice to have a person automatically committed or treated.
5. No social sanctions, whether designated criminal, civil, or therapeutic, may be invoked in the absence of the precious right to a judicial or other independent hearing, appointed counsel, and an opportunity to confront those testifying about one's past conduct or therapeutic needs.

6. Dual interference by both the criminal and the therapeutic process is prohibited.
7. An involuntary patient shall have the right to receive treatment.
8. Any compulsory treatment must be the least required reasonably to protect society.
9. All committed persons should have direct access to appointed counsel and the right, without any interference, to petition the courts for relief.
10. Those submitting to voluntary treatment should be guaranteed that they will not be subsequently transferred to a compulsory program through administrative action.*

IMPLICATIONS FOR NURSING PRACTICE

The nurse's role in psychiatric settings has ranged from custodial keeper of the keys to skilled therapeutic agent. In any of these roles, the nurse has the power to influence and determine, in part, the patient's course of treatment, since she observes and interacts with him. Nurses in all specialties have such influence, to some extent, but in the mental health field it takes on special significance because the illness is tied to behavioral symptoms. The mental health nurse, like all other members of the staff, has her own attitudes and value system, which affect her definitions of mental illness and mental health. These attitudes and values become a factor in encounters with patients. For example, the field of psychiatry has, on paper, changed its concept of homosexuality. The fact remains, however, that mental health workers in this country are members of the larger society, which for the most part has had and continues to have deeply ingrained negative attitudes toward homosexuality. Another ingrained attitude that reflects membership in the culture is the double standard of mental health for men and women, and the differences parallel the sex role stereotypes prevalent in our society.[47]

Once a person enters the mental health system as a patient, the nurse becomes a major source of information regarding his behavior. This is especially so in inpatient settings where longer contacts can occur between nurse and patient and where the nursing staff is the only group to work a 24-hour day. Many decisions regarding treatment occur in team meetings, and the nurse affects the discussion by either providing information or withholding it. If she provides information, what she reports and how she says it influence the perceptions of the patient by others. In Rosenhan's classic study, pseudopatients gained admission to

---

*Reprinted with permission from Kittrie NN: *The Right to Be Different*. Baltimore: Johns Hopkins University Press, 1971.

mental hospitals by saying they heard voices. Once admitted, they found themselves indelibly labeled with the diagnosis of schizophrenia, in spite of their subsequent normal behavior. They kept field notes for the research project and the nurses charted that these "patients" engaged in "compulsive writing." Only the other patients suspected that these pseudopatients were not mentally ill and were there for other reasons. The staff was unable to acknowledge normal behavior within the hospital milieu. In such a setting, staff members tend to see pathology more than they see normal behavior.[48]

Another potential problem with ethical dimensions that adds to the larger problem of behavior control has to do with whether nurses take the patient seriously. Does the diagnosis of mental illness affect our attitudes toward this category of persons in ways that do not allow us to take seriously what the patient says or does? Because someone is "crazy," it may be easier to dismiss him by not putting any stock in what he communicates, since it does not reflect reality. Such an attitude may be supported by the reward system of the institution where the nurse works as an employee. Not being taken seriously also occurs in situations where adults interact with children.

The medical literature discusses the ethical dilemmas arising from a paternalistic attitude that physicians have toward patients. Such an attitude tends to reduce the adult patient to the status of a child and permits the physician to violate the patient's rights, such as the right to participate in the decision-making process that influences his own welfare. Paternalism is interference with a person's liberty of action with the exclusive justification that it is for the welfare, good, happiness, needs, interests, or values of the person being coerced. Some think that self-protection or the prevention of harm to others is a sufficient warrant; however, as stated earlier, the mental health field lacks tools for predicting dangerousness. Others think that the individual's own good is never a sufficient warrant for the exercise of compulsion either by the society as a whole or by its individual members. Currently few theorists are willing to defend the "old" type of paternalism in which health professionals imposed their own values and wills upon patients. Patient autonomy is now thought to be extremely valuable and has been given great moral value. A concern is that this claim for autonomy is being used to justify a new form of paternalism.[49]

All nurses in all settings can interfere with a patient's liberty of action. Mental health nurses are in a particularly good position to do so, since either the patient has sought help with his behavioral problems and this can be interpreted as giving license to staff members to make decisions for his own good, or the patient has been committed by legal procedures and this certainly can be interpreted as giving the staff the right and obligation to interfere with the patient's liberty of action.

The ideas discussed above—namely, influencing decision making regarding mental status and treatment, not taking the patient seriously, and paternalism—can play a part in discussions of using techniques of behavior control. Nurses participate in individual and group psychotherapy as well as in behavior modification programs. Nurses also have a great influence on decisions about drugs, such as type, dosage, and frequency. One often finds in the literature, either explicitly or implicitly, the idea that drugs make the patient more amenable to other types of therapy, such as psychotherapy. Drugs also make the patient more manageable from a nursing point of view, and this raises some ethical issues around the problem of the double-agent role.

All the ethical dilemmas raised in the preceding section involve and affect the nurse. To the extent that she or he is aware of them, the nurse can examine these situations not only from a clinical perspective but also from an ethical one.

The mental health field sometimes tends to promise more than it can deliver, given the knowledge and technology it has available. This in itself raises ethical problems and dilemmas. The technology that is available has potential for abuse with regard to behavior control. The single most important factor in the intelligent use of such techniques is an ethically grounded clinician, who for moral reasons hesitates in order to think through the clinical and ethical implications of his or her actions.

One concern that must be noted here is the paucity of articles on psychiatric–mental health issues and ethics. This lack is evidenced in both the bioethics literature and the nursing literature. One article in the nursing literature researched the patterns of ethical decision making found among psychiatric nurses in inpatient settings.[50] While neither bioethics or nursing literature, the book *Psychiatry and Ethics* deals with such topics as the value dimensions of mental illness and mental health, informed consent, coercion in commitment and therapy, behavior control therapies, custodial care, and deinstitutionalization.[51]

In a society the heroes are consensually validated representations of particular values and social ideals. Our choice of heroes reflects something about the morality of our nation. A recent survey reports that American college students rank in order their heroes as Clint Eastwood and Sylvester Stallone, both of whom do acts of murder and violence in their film roles.[52] All our ethical concerns about behavior control exist in a society in which the nation's youth selects these heroes.

REFERENCES

1. Klerman GL: Behavior control and the limits of reform. *Hastings Cent Rep* August 1975.
2. Goffman E: *Asylums*. New York: Doubleday; 1961.

3. Grob GN: *Mental Institutions in America: Social Policy to 1875*. New York: Free Press; 1973.
4. Rothman DJ: *The Discovery of the Asylum: Social Order and Disorder in the New Republic*. Boston: Little, Brown; 1971.
5. Stanton AH, Schwartz MS: *The Mental Hospital*. New York: Basic Books; 1954.
6. Greenblatt M, Levinson DJ, Williams R: *The Patient and the Mental Hospital*. Glencoe, IL: Free Press; 1958.
7. Caudill WA: *A Psychiatric Hospital as a Small Society*. Cambridge, MA: Harvard University Press; 1958.
8. Greenblatt M, Levinson DJ, Klerman GL: *Mental Patients in Transition*. Springfield, IL: Charles C. Thomas; 1961.
9. Jones M: *The Therapeutic Community*. New York: Basic Books; 1953.
10. Jones M: *Beyond the Therapeutic Community*. New Haven: Yale University Press; 1968.
11. Szasz TS: *The Myth of Mental Illness*. New York: Harper & Row; 1974.
12. Boyers R, Orrill R: *R.D. Laing and Anti-Psychiatry*. New York: Harper & Row; 1971.
13. London P: *Behavior Control*. New York: Harper & Row; 1970.
14. Orwell G: *1984*. New York: Harcourt, Brace; 1959.
15. Condon R: *The Manchurian Candidate*. New York: McGraw-Hill; 1959.
16. Huxley A: *Brave New World*. New York: Harper & Row; 1932.
17. Koestler A: *Darkness at Noon*. New York: Bantam; 1970.
18. Appel W: *Cults in America: Programmed for Paradise*. New York: Henry Holt; 1985.
19. Kittrie NN: *The Right to Be Different*. Baltimore: Johns Hopkins University Press; 1971.
20. Becker HS: *Outsiders: Studies in the Sociology of Deviance*. New York: Free Press; 1963.
21. Position statement on the question of adequacy of treatment. *Am J Psychiatry*, 124:1458–1460, May 1967.
22. Roth LH: Dangerousness: In the eye of the beholder? *Am J Psychiatry*, 138:995, 1981.
23. Shah SA: Dangerousness and mental illness: Some conceptual, prediction and policy dilemmas. In Fredericks CJ (ed): *Dangerous Behavior: A Problem in Law and Mental Health*. Government Printing Office; 1978:pp 153–191.
24. Steadman HJ: The right not to be a false positive: Problems in the application of the dangerousness standard. *Psychiatry Q* 52:84–99, February 1980.
25. Steadman HJ, Morrissey JP: The statistical prediction of violent behavior: Measuring the costs of a public protectionist versus a civil liberatarian model. *Law Hum Behav* 5:263–264, April 1981.
26. Monahan J: The prediction of violent behavior: Toward a second generation of theory and policy. *Am J Psychiatry* 141:10–15, January 1984.
27. Steadman HJ: A situational approach to violence. *Int J Law Psychiatry* 5:171–186, May 1982.
28. Fisher A: *Dangerousness: Construction of an Identity*, doctoral dissertation. University of California, San Francisco, 1989.
29. Gaylin W: On the border of persuasion: A psychoanalytic look at coercion. *Psychiatry* 37:1–9, February 1974.

30. Stolz SB: *Ethical Issues in Behavior Modification.* San Francisco: Jossey-Bass; 1978.
31. Burgess A: *Clockwork Orange.* New York: Norton; 1963.
32. Augenstein L: *Come, Let Us Play God.* New York: Harper & Row; 1969.
33. Skinner BF: *Walden Two.* New York: Macmillan; 1948.
34. Skinner BF: *Science and Human Behavior.* New York: Macmillan; 1953.
35. Rogers CR: Persons or science: A philosophical question. *Am Psychol* 10:267–278, 1955.
36. Rogers CR: Implications of recent advances in prediction and behavior control. *Teachers Coll Bull* 57:316–322, 1956.
37. Rogers CR, Skinner BF: Some issues concerning the control of human behavior. *Science* 124:1057–1066, 1956.
38. Jourard S: I–thou relationship versus manipulation in counseling and psychotherapy. *J. Indiv Psychol* 15:174–179, 1959.
39. Jourard S: On the problem of reinforcement by the psychotherapist of healthy behavior in the patient. In Shaw FJ (ed): *Behavioristic Approaches to Counseling and Psychotherapy.* University, AL: University of Alabama Press; 1961.
40. Mark VH, Ervin FR: *Violence and the Brain.* New York: Harper & Row; 1970.
41. Mark VH, Neville R: Brain surgery in aggressive epileptics: Social and ethical implications. *JAMA* 238:765–772, November 12, 1973.
42. Kesey K: *One Flew Over the Cukoo's Nest.* New York: Viking; 1962.
43. Klerman GL: Psychotropic hedonism vs. pharmacological Calvinism. *Hastings Cent Rep* 2:1–3, September 1972.
44. Doudera AE, Swazey JP (eds): *Refining Treatment in Mental Health Institutions.* Ann Arbor, MI: AVPHA Press; 1982.
45. Clayton EW: From Rogers to Rivers: The rights of the mentally ill to refuse medication. *Am J Law Med* 13:7–52, 1987.
46. Kittrie NN: *The Right to Be Different,* pp 400–408.
47. Broverman IK, Broverman RD, Clarkson PS et al: Sex role stereotypes in clinical judgments of mental health. *J Consult Clin Psychol* 34:1–7, 1970.
48. Rosenhan DL: On being sane in insane places. *Science* 167:250–258, January 19, 1973.
49. Strasser M: The new paternalism. *Bioethics* 2:103–117, April 1988.
50. Garritson SH: Ethical decision making patterns. *J Psychosoc Nurs Ment Health Serv* 26:25–29, April 1988.
51. Edwards RB (ed): *Psychiatry and Ethics.* Buffalo, NY: Prometheus; 1982.
52. Fink PJ: Presidential address: On being ethical in an unethical world. *Am J Psychiatry* 146:1097–1104, September 1989.

CHAPTER 11

Mental Retardation

ETHICAL DILEMMAS

Any discussion of ethical dilemmas and the mentally retarded must take into account the concept of respect for persons. Private morality concerns itself with respecting the distinctive human endowment as we find it in ourselves, whereas public morality is concerned with respecting the distinctive human endowment as we find it in others. Private and public morality therefore represent two aspects of a single, fundamental moral principle.[1,2] We feel brotherly love, agape, respect toward thóse regarded as persons. This notion leaves open the possibility of debate as to who or what properly and truly constitutes a person we are to regard with respect. Traditionally, it has been assumed that basic to the distinctive endowment of a human being is his ability to reason. Kant, a typical and supreme representative of the Age of Enlightenment, developed the thesis that possession of a rational will is the quality that gives a person absolute worth.[3] Rational will is the quality of the generic self, or the distinctive endowment of a human being that is respected for no other reason than that the individual is a human person. Kant's thesis has influenced directly or indirectly our attitudes toward a number of groups, including the mentally retarded.

The concept of a *person* is already an evaluative concept with something of the force of "that which makes a human being valuable" implied in it. But the questions remain: Why do we respect or value a person? What makes a human being a person?[4] In the field of developmental disability, as we move along the continuum from borderline retarded, do we perceive each individual as a person or do we draw the line based on moral reasoning ability and think only of some on the continuum as persons we respect? If personhood is *not* dependent on moral reasoning ability, what is it that indicates that someone is a person and what is it about persons that requires our respect?

For many individuals, the term *person* refers to a cluster of features beyond rationality, having a self-concept, and being conceived by humans.[5] Other features of personhood seem to include *biological factors* (descended from humans; having a certain genetic make-up; having a head, hands, arms, eyes; capable of locomotion, breathing, eating, and sleeping), *psychological factors* (having a concept of self and of one's interests and desires; the ability to use language or symbol systems), *rationality factors* (the ability to reason and draw conclusions; the ability to learn from past experiences), *social factors* (the ability to work in groups; the ability to recognize and consider the interests of others; the abilities to love and sympathize), and *legal factors* (the ability to own property and inherit goods; being subject to the law and protected by it; citizenship). This is not a list of necessary and sufficient conditions for personhood but simply features that are more or less typical of those who are referred to as "persons."

If individuals lack some of the above mentioned biological, psychological, and rationality factors, are they less qualified as persons? Is respect for them as persons dependent on which factors are present and which are lacking? Or do individuals merely need to be members of the human community to be counted as persons? Respect for them is then dependent on whether or not the community values them and accords them full rights and responsibilities as members of the community. Our position in the personhood debate is that human embodiment with the capacity for consciousness or social interaction (or both) constitutes a "person," that persons have rights and responsibilities, and that persons have a moral claim on other members of the community.[6] Mentally retarded and physically disabled individudals are worthy of our respect simply because they are persons. The focus of concern is thus how society fulfills its duties and obligations to safeguard the basic rights of the mentally retarded and physically disabled individuals when they cannot, by virtue of their retardation or disabilities, completely do so themselves.

Crocker and Cushna, for example, outline the "normal rights" of the mentally retarded that must be defended as including the right to family living, educational opportunities, treatment and habilitation services, employment, support in the development of contracts, and confidentiality in personal records. They also outline "special rights" as including qualified advocacy and guardianship capacity; protection against use of drugs and behavior modification techniques, including experimental procedures; counseling and safeguards regarding reproduction; and intelligent exposure to life situations involving risk.[7]

Friedman, on the other hand, outlines the rights of mentally retarded persons according to whether they reside in an institution or in the community. Mentally retarded persons in institutions should be recognized as having the right to habilitation and the right to protection from harm; freedom from hazardous, intrusive, and experimental procedures; the right to sexual expression; the right to fair compensation for institutional labor; the right to a humane physical and psychological environment; the right to dignity and privacy, religious freedom, behavioral and leisure-time activities; and prompt and appropriate medical treatment consistent with the accepted standards of medical practice in the community.[8] Mentally retarded persons in the community should be recognized as having the right to education; the right to reside in the community; sexual and marital rights; the right to a barrier-free environment; employment rights; the right to be free from discrimination in voting, driving, and other rights of citizenship; the right to medical care; and the right to participate in federal financial assistance and other benefit programs.[9]

The rights of the mentally retarded have not been so broadly interpreted and accepted, however. Consider, for example, the abuse through involuntary sterilization of many mentally retarded individuals throughout United States' history.[10] The notorious 1927 United States Supreme Court decision upholding a State of Virginia statute to allow the sterilization of 18-year-old Carrie Buck and other more recent decisions make us realize that the rights of the mentally retarded have often been abrogated.[11] The federal government no longer authorizes the use of federal funds to sterilize the mentally incompetent or anyone under 21 years of age.

One aspect of the sterilization argument concerns the parameters of governmental control. No one, whether a critic or an advocate of regulation, believes that anyone should ever be coerced into accepting sterilization. Advocates of regulation believe that abuses occur frequently enough, especially with vulnerable groups such as minors, the poor, and the mentally imcompetent, to warrant strong controls. Critics of such regulations do not believe such abuse is the case and maintain that some, including the poor and the mentally incompetent, have actually been abused by being denied sterilization by the arbitrary judgments of a physician or hospital. This moral dilemma raises the question as to whether any of the mentally retarded should be sterilized, and, if so, which ones, on what grounds, and on whose consent shall it be done? Some believe that sterilization ought to be available for people who are sexually active but unable to care for a child. Others believe that only the mentally retarded capable of giving informed consent should ever be candidates for sterilization.[12,13]

Since the ethical dilemmas of informed consent in research have been discussed elsewhere, the problem of mentally retarded individuals participating in research studies will be mentioned only briefly here. As indicated, certain groups, such as the mentally ill, children, prisoners, and the mentally retarded, present special problems as research subjects because of the informed consent requirement and the possibility of coercion. The famous Willowbrook Study, conducted on mentally retarded institutionalized children, raised numerous ethical questions about the use of vulnerable populations in research studies.[14] Public discussion about the study helped create new guidelines for the informed consent of children and the mentally retarded in research studies. At issue was the ethics of undertaking research on institutionalized individuals when the research is neither therapeutic nor likely to benefit the individual research subjects and may not benefit other people in the future.[15-18]

In summary, the ethical dilemmas discussed with regard to the mentally retarded can be listed as concerning the concept of *person*; how we define mental retardation and the consequences this definition has; problems encountered by the mentally retarded in institutions and in the community regarding their rights; and the moral reasoning that society uses in balancing its resources and values to determine the risks and benefits for the individual and for society itself.

GENERAL BACKGROUND INFORMATION

The concept of developmental disability recognizes mental retardation, regardless of cause, as a facet within a spectrum of possible abnormalities.[19] The Congress enacted Public Law 91-517 in 1970, defining developmental disability as:

> ... a disability attributable to mental retardation, cerebral palsy, epilepsy, or another neurological condition of an individual found by the Secretary to be closely related to mental retardation or to require treatment similar to that required for mentally retarded individuals, which disability originates before such individual attains age 18, which has continued or can be expected to continue indefinitely, and which constitutes a substantial handicap to such individual.

Not as specific as it might be, this definition does, however, recognize disorders of adjustment, communication, locomotion, and intellectual function and emphasizes the generally nonprogressive nature and irreversibility of these disabilities.

The Developmentally Disabled Assistance and Bill of Rights Act, Public Law 94-103, which became law in October of 1975, broadened the definition of developmental problems and the strategies for strengthening services and safeguarding individual rights. This act authorized grants for the purpose of developing services and training personnel and established a National Advisory Council on Services and Facilities for the Developmentally Disabled. The American Association on Mental Deficiency states that the term "mental retardation" refers to significantly subaverage general intellectual functioning existing concurrently with deficits in adaptive behavior and manifested during the developmental period.

Mental retardation, ultimately a social attribute, comprises at least three components: organic, functional, and social. The organic component we refer to as impairment, the functional component as disability, and the social component as handicap. Epidemiological understanding of any disorder will differ depending on which of the three components is counted. In mild mental retardation, the rule is the absence of recognized impairment but the presence of functional disability measured in terms of an IQ below a given point. The extent of social handicap varies with age and social setting.

Unfortunately, occasionally the social role of mental handicap has been conferred on a person with neither brain impairment nor functional disability. In this country and in England there have been reported cases of individuals with IQs within the normal range being placed in institutions for the retarded and so acquiring the social role of mental retardation.[20]

Incidence measures the frequency with which disorders arise anew in a population during a specific period of time. Incidence rates in mental retardation must often obtain their data from cases clinically identified on entry to health services, and therefore we have only approximations, for two reasons. In these situations, entry into the health services for the mentally retarded rarely coincides with the onset of the disorder. Furthermore, all who have the disorder may not be represented in the sample, since all mentally retarded people may not be health service consumers. Prevalence describes a disorder existing in a population at one particular time. It ignores the time of disorder onset and, especially in chronic disorders, it limits the inferences connecting cause and effect. Incidence gives the best view of the circumstances in which disorders arise over a period of time in a population but depends on usage of services. Prevalence gives a good view of the needs of a specific population, such as the mentally retarded, at a given time and is also less dependent on service usage.[21]

Although prevalence rates of mental retardation have been confounded both by definition variations of mental retardation and by the differing assessments of coexisting impairment in an individual, it has been estimated that in the United States, 3 percent of the general population, or 6.1 million people, have IQs of less than 70. Each year between 100,000 and 200,000 of the babies born join this group. Of the total, about 2.4 million are children and minors under 21 years of age. About 2.1 million of these children could be classified as mildly retarded, 144,000 as moderately retarded, and 120,000 as severely retarded.[22] In this country, admission records from large medical centers for children show that 25 to 30 percent of all these admissions have been for genetic disease, mental retardation, or congenital malformations.[23] Experts have recently catalogued almost 2000 autosomal dominant, recessive, and sex-linked disorders, but even more exist since they omitted a large number of polygenically inherited disorders.[24] These data would support the notion that few families remain untouched by genetic disorder, the results of which can range from mild to severe retardation.

The etiological classification of mental retardation can be divided into two overall categories, genetic and acquired. The genetic category contains such examples as Down's syndrome, a chromosomal abnormality; phenylketonuria, a disorder of amino acid metabolism; and Tay-Sachs, a disorder of lipid metabolism, to mention only a few conditions. Examples of acquired mental retardation can be further categorized into (1) prenatal, when infection such as rubella, toxin effects, and placental insufficiency occur; (2) perinatal, when prematurity, anoxia, or cerebral damage occur; (3) postnatal, when brain injury, infection such as meningitis, anoxia, effects of poison, and sociocultural factors such as deprivation occur. The examples given here do not exhaust the possibilities but serve to give some idea of the complexities of mental retardation.

From 1967 through 1974, Dr. Allen Crocker, Director of the Development Evaluation Clinic, Children's Hospital, Boston, collected data on diagnostic classifications by apparent mechanism. In a total sample of 1058 mentally retarded children, he found 34 percent due to early influences on embyronic development, 27 percent due to unknown causes, 19 percent due to environmental and social problems, 11 percent due to other pregnancy problems and perinatal morbidity, 5 percent due to heredity issues, and 4 percent due to acquired childhood diseases. The exact cause of mental retardation in many cases can be most difficult to elucidate. The difficulty becomes compounded by genetic and environmental interaction, prematurity, low birth weight, and perinatal complications. The causes of mental retardation and other developmental disabilities overlap and are inextricably related in complex ways. It has been estimated that nongenetic factors may contribute as much as one half of the total variance in IQ scores.[25] A detailed presentation of the causes and prevalence of mental retardation remains beyond the scope of this chapter. These remarks serve only to indicate the magnitude and complexities of the problem, to set the stage for a discussion of other aspects of mental retardation, and to provide basic information for ethical reasoning. If the reader wishes additional material on what might be called the more biological dimensions, the *Mental Retardation Abstracts* will be an invaluable reference. Also, any number of books as well as papers in professional journals have been published on the topic.

HISTORICAL BACKGROUND

In the United States before 1810, the majority of the mentally ill and retarded lived in homes with their families or friends or, if without a social network, they could be found in poorhouses and jails. The era of the Industrial Revolution, which brought with it waves of immigrants and a beginning shift from a rural society to an urban one, defined deviant behavior as a product of the social, political, and economic environment of the time. Social reformers viewed this environment as chaotic, disordered, and lacking stability. The traditional social procedures and institutions were breaking down and in some case dissolving. This situation in turn created great societal stresses and strains.[26] From Europe at about this time, news came of cures for insanity and deviant behavior, with emphasis on humane care in special residential institutions. This "moral treatment" developed along with the increasing belief in the physical base of certain deviant behaviors. Within this context, individuals exhibiting these behaviors became the legitimate concern of physiology and medicine.[27] By 1860, 28 of the then 33 states had built public institutions to house and care for this segment of the population. This growth in institutional care, occurring mostly between 1830 and the 1850s, became defined as the most proper treatment method.[28]

This era, which emphasized the social origins of disease, also defined idiocy and feeblemindedness as social problems. Major reformers of the day had their ideas applied to a large extent because they fitted the pervading assumptions about the therapeutic effects of institutionalization. And so the transformation of these institutions from residential schools to custodial asylums had support from the society at large, as well as from the professionals who ran them. One writer maintains that these professionals did not necessarily invent the concept of the "menace of the feebleminded," but they did support its propagation, benefited from it, and until the 1920s opposed alternatives to residential segregation.[29] Essentially, the patterns of development in the institutions for the mentally retarded paralleled those used in the treatment of other forms of dependency and deviancy.

These larger social changes also had an impact on the educational system of the country. Society increasingly called on schools to train for economic, social, and civic roles, and in assuming these functions the school became the primary defender of the social order. By the 1920s, the experts and the general public assumed that by making an educational problem out of any social problem it could be effectively treated.[30] Other changes in the educational system affecting the mentally retarded also occurred during these years. The adoption of a corporate-industrial model of educational organization—in which the administration became managers, teachers the workers, the curriculum the technology, and the students the raw material for processing,[31]—combined with a rise in vocationalism that led to a definition of equality of educational opportunity,[32] and the development of intelligence testing[33] affected the role of the school vis-à-vis the mentally retarded. These changes, occurring in the first three decades of this century, combined to provide a major impetus to the emergence of special education for the mentally handicapped.

The special education movement, although gathering support from various groups, never achieved the full public acceptance enjoyed by the earlier asylum movement.[34] A variety of reasons accounted for the lack of acceptance, one of which was parental hostility that was kept in play by the school's failure to distinguish among the different categories of children—that is, the mentally retarded, the behaviorally disruptive, the physically handicapped, and the truant children. In short, these special classes became the dumping grounds for children whom, because it lacked ways of accommodating them, the educational system could not tolerate.[35] However, an even more central problem persisted well into the latter half of this century, when special education experienced a substantial growth. The original assumption underlying the special education concept remained unquestioned. The results of this central problem can best be described by employing W.I. Thomas's famous aphorism, "If men define the situation as real, then it is real in its consequences." That is to say, with regard to the mentally retarded, once a given individual's situation becomes defined, whether accurately or inaccurately, this definition becomes "the truth," which others use as the basis for their relations with that individual. The continued emphasis on IQ as an irremedial constant remained intact and effectively undercut the significance of psychological and cultural variables. This lead to what Blatt calls "a predeterministic mental set," with fatalistic overtones. Education assumed that a lack of competence in traditional school requirements could be equated with a lack of competence in other areas of social activity.[36] The phenomenon of segregation for the mentally retarded in educational settings interacted with the concern over mislabeling a child as mentally retarded when in fact he was not. However, the basic assumption that the expected benefits of categorizing and labeling children always outweighed the disadvantages went unchallenged.

THE EFFECTS OF LABELING

The range of intellectual capabilities demonstrated by individuals labeled as mentally retarded varies greatly and can be divided into five categories: borderline, IQ 68 to 85; mild, IQ 52 to 67; moderate, IQ 36 to 51; severe, IQ 20 to 35; and profound, IQ under 20. The enormous and complex ramifications of this labeling process and the consequences of labeling will be discussed only briefly. Begab distinguishes between classification and labeling, related but differing processes, since each has a distinctive purpose and use.[37] Classification systems, designed primarily to provide statistical data about groups of similar individuals or cases, furnish the basis for measuring incidence, prevalence, characteristics, and other information, including the success of programs established to prevent or ameliorate the condition.[38] Such a procedure as classification has many problems. The most basic problem stems from the difficulty of any effort to categorize the totality and complexity of a human being. No matter how multidimensional the classification methods, their imperfections and inadequacies will soon become apparent. An interesting paradox that compounds this serious problem in classifying any group can be noted. The more knowledge science develops about a given entity, in this case mental retardation, the more difficult classification becomes because of the additional dimensions and complexities. The classification system presents special problems in dealing with individuals in the mild or moderate categories. Frequent discrepancies occur between adaptive behavior and measured intelligence, making it difficult to determine who should be classified in which category. These problems may be further compounded by the sociopolitical processes at play in the society at any given time. For example, in recent years, questions have been raised about the use of IQ testing as a basis for classifying and placing individuals in programs. The limitations of IQ tests and the possible errors in using them point to their disadvantage as the only source of information used to classify people. Other problems can be identified, including the presumed-cultural-bias controversy[39] and the difficulty in assessing social competence. The IQ and social competence tests must be supplemented by life history data, biomedical information, and clinical judgment.

Classification would not be possible without the labeling process. The label of mental retardation, like all such labels, serves as a shorthand way of saying a number of things about an individual or group. Although labels may be necessary to facilitate communication, they do tend to conjure up stereotypes, especially socially defined pejorative ones, of the labeled person. For example, people hold an image of the alcoholic as a skid-row bum and not as the business executive, although in this latter group alcoholism constitutes a problem of some magnitude. Labels are not inherently bad, although they can, and sometimes do, come in for abuse. With the mental retardation label, one abuse derives from overlooking the vast range of individual differences found in the people so labeled. This abuse can lead us to interact with all mentally retarded persons as if no differences existed. All of us, including the mentally retarded, gain and maintain our concept of self from interaction with others. If we constantly respond to a retarded individual in stereotyped ways, he continually receives feedback about himself that may be based more on our preconceptions and stereotypes than on the individual himself. This could lead to a self-fulfilling prophecy, in that the mentally retarded person begins to respond to us on the basis of our notion of him. For example, if we view him as dependent and unable to do for himself, then he may behave to fit this view of him. The labeling concept in mental retardation remains complex, and the voluminous literature on the topic does not always provide us with conclusive data regarding the multiple dimensions of the process.[40-45] Although some believe this process causes great harm by stigmatizing, others point out that once labeled accurately, a mentally retarded individual has access to beneficial services. Perhaps it will help if we remember that the mental retardation label is the most stigmatizing of all in our society.[46]

ATTITUDES TOWARD THE RETARDED

One of the central concerns regarding the mental retardation label is the attitude that society holds toward this population. The social context out of which the label comes reflects the attitudes that also in large part determine society's reaction to the mentally retarded. Major attention has been given to the negative consequences of classifying and labeling children as mentally retarded. These studies have tended to search for evidence to illustrate the nature and manifestations of stigma, without examining possible beneficial consequences of the classification system.[47]

The rationale for research on attitudes toward the retarded, or any other deviant population, rests on the assumption that when a society has more favorable attitudes toward such a group, more enlightened treatment of them ensues. The other side of this assumption, negative attitudes that lead to the group remaining in a more unenviable societal position than necessary, has been documented. In an era such as our own, when the emphasis has shifted to keeping the retarded in the community by having them participate in community-based programs, the attitudes of and acceptance by the local residents become a crucial factor in the success or failure of such an endeavor. As part of this change, some school systems have abolished their segregated special classes and have reintegrated the mentally retarded students into the regular school classes. The general idea of integration takes into account the student's ability to handle the situation and the existence of separate programs as needed. For example, a plan may include integration for social and nonacademic portions of the curriculum with special teaching in resource programs. This concept of integration does not imply that such programs for the mentally retarded would be to the detriment of more competent students.

The general public views the retarded person as a mongoloid or a brain-damaged individual.[48] This view persists among the public, although professionals in the field know that the overwhelming proportion of retardation can be attributed to cultural or environmental differences and not to organic or genetic abnormalities. Patterns have emerged from numerous community attitude surveys. The public has more favorable attitudes toward the mildly mentally retarded than toward the severely retarded. They often confuse mental retardation with mental illness and show a general ignorance regarding the retarded themselves and the services available to them.[49] In addition, the neurologically disabled (e.g, cerebral palsy and aphasia) may be both mislabeled and misunderstood as mentally retarded because of their functional disabilities. Research does not consistently indicate that contact with retarded people results in more favorable attitudes toward them.[50-52]

The research on peer attitudes, relying in the main on sociometric instruments, shows the response to mildly retarded children in the school system. A number of studies demonstrate that regardless of the particular educational model employed, educable mentally retarded children are not so well accepted by their peers as are nonretarded children.[53-55] One study indicated that peer groups accepted the educable mentally retarded from a higher socioeconomic status better than they did those from a lower status.[56] Another study concluded that special or regular class placement does not affect the neighborhood interaction patterns of retarded children, since the other children ignore them regardless of placement.[57]

Little research has been conducted on the attitudes of those health professionals most likely to come into contact with the mentally retarded. Studies on the attitudes of school teachers have been undertaken that may throw some light on one aspect of the immediate future, when more retarded children will attend regular classrooms. Studies show that regular education teachers do not have especially positive attitudes toward children with a mental retardation label[58] and the length of teaching experience either does not promote positive changes in attitudes[59] or results in more unfavorable attitudes.[60] Numerous studies have documented the fact that a primary function of educational institutions has become the allocation of persons to adult roles and statuses in the larger society.[61-64] The attitudes of teachers, which have been shown to have a significant effect on children's academic performance,[65] take on special meaning within this context. The extent to which teachers' attitudes or expectations affect retarded children's performance remains open to question, but they may influence his social status among his peer group, if nothing else.[66]

In the past, the school nurse has encountered the mildly retarded child in the school system. At present, the trend is toward accommodating the more severely and multiply handicapped with physical and mental disability in the public school system. Until recently, these children would have been either in a day-care program or in no program at all. So the role of the school vis-à-vis this population will grow in importance. In addition, now that this trend will keep the mentally retarded out of total institutions, they will seek medical services in the general hospital as needed. Therefore, the hospital nurse is more likely to have contact with this group than in the past. These changes have occurred within the newly expanded legal and civil rights for the mentally retarded.

THE LEGAL AND CIVIL RIGHTS OF THE RETARDED

The interaction between the law and mental retardation presents the most confused, ambiguous picture in the entire mental health area.[67] A clearly demonstrated example of this situation can be found in the legal standard of mental retardation that serves as the threshold label invoked in statutes authorizing confinement. In at least five states, the statutes read that mental deficiency shall mean mental deficiency as defined by appropriate clinical authorities.[68] The law in these cases totally abdicates responsibility in favor of clinicians, and this may lead to the practice of unregulated admissions and the abuse of the retarded person's civil liberties. The typical statutory definition of mental deficiency uses such phrases as "incapable of managing himself and his affairs" and "for whose own welfare or that of others, supervision, guidance, care, or control is necessary or admissible."[69] These statutes recognize that the justification of confinement in these cases cannot be on the danger-to-others concept but rather must be on the idea that it benefits the retarded person, his family, or the community. The effectiveness of these statutes is limited, since most retarded individuals become confined while still minors and therefore they have no recourse to a court of law.

Murdock identified three interacting areas affecting the civil rights of the mentally retarded: guardianship, institutionalization, and education.[70] Deeply rooted in our legal system and our general notions of society lies the belief that parents are the natural guardians of children. This belief implies a compatibility of interest between parent and child and the ability on the parent's part to care for and represent the child in his dealings with the institutions of society. However, as the President's Committee on Mental Retardation points out, the provisions in most states largely consider or assume the retarded person to be without rights and deny him due process or the equal protection of the law.[71] Moreover, a conflict of interest may exist between the parent and the child. For example, the parent may be motivated to seek institutionalization for a number of reasons other than the best interests of the child himself—for example, perceived stigma of mental retardation, economic stress, physical and mental frustration, or consideration for other children in the family. The retarded child's best interest may well lie in living with his family and in the community, but theirs may not lie in keeping him.[72] The film *Who Should Survive?*[73] graphically illustrates a most fundamental conflict of interest in depicting the real-life situation where, because of the parents' decision, the hospital withheld minor corrective surgery from a Down's syndrome infant with an intestinal obstruction. The infant died a slow death from dehydration. This situation raises numerous ethical dilemmas that will be discussed in another section of this chapter.

The rights of any institutionalized person can be abused, and this may be especially true for the mentally retarded. While many rights to which the retarded are entitled have been outlined, including the right to visitation by family members at all reasonable hours,[74] the right to receive compensation for their labor,[75] and the right to normal relationships with the opposite sex,[76] probably the most crucial rights for this group are the right to a humane physical and psychological environment and the right to adequate treatment. The need for judicial recognition of constitutional standards with respect to the care of the institutionalized retarded arose from abuses of these rights, many of which have been documented in legal testimony.

The genesis of a legally enforceable right to treatment concept appeared in a 1960 article advocating the rights of the mentally ill, but the mentally retarded were not mentioned.[77] The first significant judicial development occurred in 1966 when the District of Columbia court determined that the 1964 Hospitalization of the Mentally Ill Act did provide a right to treatment, which could be judicially enforced.[78]

Subsequent court decisions have further defined the right to treatment and have expanded it to include a constitutional right to the "least restrictive alternative." This means that when someone becomes ill and in need of treatment but is not dangerous to himself or others, he cannot legally be confined in the most restrictive setting, such as a locked hospital ward. The rationale for this principle is that "commitment entails an extraordinary deprivation of liberty" and that "such a drastic curtailment of the rights of citizens must be narrowly, even grudgingly, constructed in order to avoid deprivation of liberty without due process of law."[79] Not until 1972, when the third decision in the *Wyatt v Stickney* case mentioned the right to habilitation for the mentally retarded, did this group receive consideration. The court defined habilitation as the "the process by which the staff of the institution assists the resident to acquire and maintain those life skills which enable him to cope more effectively with the demands on his own person and of his environment and to raise the level of his physical, mental, and social efficiency."[80] Habilitation, although not limited to such programs, includes programs of formal structured education and treatment. This has extended the right to treatment in medical terms to include education. Further refinement of this concept encompassed the nature of the living conditions generally—whether each patient has an individualized plan and generally enjoys a humane psychological and physical environment.

Although the 1969 President's Committee on Mental Retardation estimated that approximately 60 percent of the retarded school age children were not receiving an education,[81] Murdock maintains that the prospects for the retarded appear the highest in the area of education. He bases his statement on several factors. A federal constitutional basis for arguing that the retarded are entitled to a public education now exists. In addition, many state constitutions require the establishment of a public educational system open to all. The requirement of upgrading the quality of habilitation in state institutions and the concomitant resulting cost spiral creates tremendous pressures to provide services to the retarded outside of the traditional, huge, warehouse-like institutions.[82]

To expect the judiciary to correct all the wrongs experienced by the mentally retarded is a quixotic notion, but recent events in the legal system have opened the courtroom door to the advocates of the retarded. In this process, the American public has had an opportunity to gain insight into the dimensions, including the legal and ethical ones, involved in caring for the retarded children and adults in our society.

The United Nations General Assembly in 1971 adopted a declaration on the rights of the retarded that reads:

> Reaffirming faith in human rights and fundamental freedoms and in the principles of peace, of the dignity and worth of the human person and of social justice proclaimed in the Charter,
>
> Recalling the principles of the Universal Declaration of Human Rights, the International Covenants on Human Rights, the Declaration of the Rights of the Child and the standards already set for social programs in the Constitutions, conventions, accommodations and resolutions of the International Labour Organization, the United Nations Educational, Scientific and Cultural Organization, the World Health Organization, the United Nations Children's Fund and of other organizations concerned,
>
> Emphasizing that the Declaration on Social Progress and Development has proclaimed the necessity of protecting the rights and assuring the welfare and rehabilitation of the physically and mentally disadvantaged,
>
> Bearing in mind the necessity of assisting mentally retarded persons to develop their abilities in various fields of activities and of promoting their integration as far as possible in normal life,
>
> Aware that certain countries, at their present stage of development, can devote only limited efforts to this end,
>
> Proclaims this Declaration on the Rights of Mentally Retarded Persons and calls for national and international action to ensure that it will be used as a common basis and frame of reference for the protection of these rights:

1. The mentally retarded person has, to the maximum degree of feasibility, the same rights as other human beings.
2. The mentally retarded person has a right to proper medical care and physical therapy and to such education, training, rehabilitation and guidance as will enable him to develop his ability and maximum potential.
3. The mentally retarded person has a right to economic security and to a decent standard of living. He has a right to perform productive work or to engage in any other meaningful occupation to fullest possible extent of his capabilities.
4. Whenever possible, the mentally retarded person should live with his own family or with foster parents and participate in different forms of community life. The family with which he lives should receive assistance. If care in an institution becomes necessary, it should be provided in surroundings and other circumstances as close as possible to those of normal life.
5. The mentally retarded person has a right to a qualified guardian when this is required to protect his personal well-being and interests.
6. The mentally retarded person has a right to protection from exploitation, abuse and degrading treatment. If prosecuted for any offense, he shall have a right to due process of law with full recognition being given to his degree of mental responsibility.
7. Whenever mentally retarded persons are unable because of the severity of their handicap to exercise all their rights in a meaningful way, or it should become necessary to restrict or deny some or all of these rights, the procedure used for that restriction or denial of rights must contain proper legal safeguards against every form of abuse. This procedure must be based on an evaluation of the social capability of the mentally retarded person by qualified experts and must be subject to periodic review and to the rights of appeal to higher authorities.

Despite broad statements of rights of the mentally retarded, individuals labeled as "mentally retarded" in the community continue to suffer infringement of a variety of rights available to nonretarded citizens. They are often denied the right to travel, the right to free association, and the right to privacy. They may also be denied the right to marry, the right to be licensed (for driving cars and for certain occupations like barbering), and the right to enter into contracts (such as buying a television on time). When institutionalized, mentally retarded individuals often experience other deprivations, such as their rights to sexual expression, education, and protection from harm. To protect the civil and legal rights of the mentally retarded, advocates for the mentally retarded find they need to rely on the Constitution of the United States, federal legislation and regulations (such as the Rehabilitation Act of 1973, the Education Act, the Developmentally Disabled Assistance and Bill of Rights Act, and the Fair Labor Standards Act), and not just statements of rights.

GENETIC SCREENING

Governments have special concerns for the health of citizens. For example, many nations have statutory programs to provide for the control of contagious diseases. There have also been times when the state legally forced a person to have treatment even when no discernible risk to society from the illness could be demonstrated. The boundaries of permissible government activities to regulate more generally the health of society as a whole have been delineated, in part, by such constitutional constraints as: the guarantee of the freedom to religious convictions; the guarantee that no person will be deprived of life, liberty, or property without due process of the law; and the guarantee that no state shall deny to any person within its jurisdiction the equal protection of the law. The doctrine of Fundamental Interests holds that certain human activities not mentioned in the Bill of Rights deserve special judicial protection. One of these activities, privacy or the right to be left alone, has slowly expanded to include rights of personal decision making.[83] No absolute and clear delineation of the outer limits of government action pursuant to the public health power can be made. The state's power to order an individual to undergo a medical procedure—such as immunization, sterilization, blood tests, and x-rays—has far-reaching implications. The potential of this power for both evil and good is obvious and any proposal for the extension of the power deserves very careful scrutiny.[84] Genetic-screening legislation represents one such extension of this power.

Genetic screening is defined as the search for those suffering from a genetically based disease or those possessing a certain genotype that may be inherited. Genetic screening may be done for several reasons: for the purpose of detecting disease; to gain reproductive information; to conduct epidemiological research.[85]

In screening for disease, the object is to discover persons with a specific disease or those who have genes that might lead to disease. Once such persons are identified, they are offered treatment to manage their disease or to reverse or prevent the adverse effects of a genetic disorder. In screening for reproductive information, the purpose is to discover persons within the population who have genes that, when joined with other genes, may lead to adverse genetic effects in offspring. The implicit assumption in this kind of screening is that persons may wish to include knowledge of their genotype and the possible risks of producing adversely affected children in their reproductive decisions. In screening for epidemiological purposes, public health authorities are monitoring the incidence of genetic disorders as a means to learning about their causes. This kind of screening may also be done for health purposes or to study the natural history of a genetic disorder for which there is currently no treatment.

The benefits of screening for communicable disorders in this country are known to many but the value of genetic screening has often been surrounded by controversy and doubt.[86] This has been due in part to the lack of specific criteria for screening programs and the lack of reliable testing materials to detect genetic disorders. These two problems are quite evident in the history of phenylketonuria (PKU) testing in the United States during the 1960s.

A diagnostic test for PKU was known in 1934 when it was discovered that the fresh urine from some mentally retarded children changed color in the presence of ferric chloride. It was later learned that children with PKU who were placed on a special diet early in life did not become mentally retarded.[87] Screening of all infants for PKU did not occur, however, until the bacterial inhibition assay for PKU was developed by Robert Guthrie in 1961.[88] PKU thus emerged as the first genetically determined condition for which there was both means of easy identification and treatment. By the mid-1960s, the majority of states passed PKU testing laws, with the result that the test is now offered in every state.

The phenomenal growth of PKU laws over a short period of time is rather interesting. Some analysts of health policy suggest that the small budget outlay required for a state PKU-testing program, combined with the unquestionable benefit of a plan to reduce mental retardation, provided special interest groups (such as the National Association for Retarded Children) with a powerful lobbying weapon that easily won support.[89] Others have suggested that it was the threat of mental retardation, not PKU per se, that impressed the state legislators to act so quickly.[90] Whatever the reasons, the growth of PKU screening and its surrounding controversies have provided important lessons that may apply to genetic screening in general.

For example, the lack of counseling and follow-up in most early state-mandated PKU testing programs demonstrated that the planning of screening and interventions for all gene-related metabolic disease must be subjected to careful analysis before being instituted. The initial testing methodology for PKU was not of uniform quality from state to state. As a result, treatment for false positive reactions produced mental retardation in otherwise normal children who were wrongly placed on the PKU diet. In addition, few states required that affected children be placed on a low-phenylalanine diet or gave statutory consideration to genetic counseling for families of affected children.[91]

Only a few states created PKU registries, a special problem for PKU-affected women now of childbearing age.[92] Successfully treated by a special diet in their early years, PKU-affected women survived child-hood with normal mentality and are bearing their own children. How-ever, if the PKU-affected woman does not go back on the low-phenylalanine diet during pregnancy, her fetus will suffer brain damage in utero as a result of the excess maternal phenylalanine. The implica-tion of this new problem is that counseling must be made available to any PKU-affected female before childbearing age and that prenatal ex-aminations should possibly include routine PKU testing of all pregnant women.

Despite numerous problems in the PKU testing experience, state genetic screening programs grew in number through the 1960s and 1970s. Screening for genetic disease was believed to be a desirable goal of society and was even emphasized in President Richard Nixon's 1971 health message to the nation. President Nixon noted the incidence of sickle cell anemia among the black population in the United States and asked the National Institutes of Health (NIH) to increase its funding for sickle cell anemia research.[93] Within a few months, reports of sickle cell anemia appeared in the national news media and there was an increase in federal funding for sickle cell anemia research. As sickle cell anemia moved to center stage in the genetic disease theater, state legislatures acted on hastily constructed sickle cell anemia screening proposals in much the same manner that they did on PKU screening proposals a few years before. By the end of 1976, other legislation had been passed related to Cooley's anemia, Tay-Sachs disease, and other genetic disor-ders.[94]

Genetic disorder legislation, designed to influence childbearing de-cisions by heterozygous couples and to reduce the number of geneti-cally defective children born, tended to overlook the dangers implicit in such laws. Because of the association of sickle cell anemia with only one race, screening laws confronted an unusual equal-protection problem. This situation became further compounded by the fact that these laws failed to provide for confidentiality of test information; availability of competent, free genetic-counseling services; and programs to edu-cate the general public about genetic disease. Similar problems encoun-tered in other disease-specific legislation, such as laws regarding Tay-Sachs disease and Cooley's anemia, raise larger questions as to the appropriateness and effectiveness of this multiplication of disease-specific laws.[95]

Genetic-screening programs have the goals of treatment and reduc-tion of the number of births of affected persons. The major traditional goal has been treatment of identified persons with a given condition; however, the other goal has increasingly received attention within the context of developing health care priorities and allocating resources. This raises a myriad of ethical issues.

At present, the government seems to favor the "pure voluntarism" model in the area of eugenic legislation. Screening legislation should be written with a clear understanding of the immediate potential risks and benefits and a recognition of policy implications. In addition, these laws should safeguard the integrity of the individual who will be tested. It is true that mandatory screening laws would possibly achieve a more rapid reduction of genetic disease than would voluntary screening; however, the unique potential that genetic data hold for subtle social and political discrimination can be viewed as a risk that outweighs the envisioned benefit.[96]

GENETIC COUNSELING

For Milunsky, the premise that human rights of personal inviolability include the fundamental right to life with a self-determined destiny and the right to marry and procreate served to establish the guiding principles in genetic counseling.[97] These rights delineate the providence of moral autonomy and individual privacy in decisions about procreation.

The World Health Organization Expert Committee on genetic counseling has endorsed the nondirective approach with parents.[98] Although this practice has been recommended, Sorenson's research points to the difficulties confronting counselors when the evidence shows that 54 percent of counselors tend to leave all decisions to parents, while 64 percent of this same group reported that they informed parents in a way that would guide them toward an "appropriate" decision.[99] The intrinsic danger involved in this paradox found in nondirective counseling, as well as in the more direct counseling approach, is the possible insinuation by the counselor of his or her own religious, racial, eugenic, or other dictates into the counseling encounter.

Capron argues that parents have a legal right to receive full information, including options, risks, benefits, and consequences available or foreseeable as they deliberate their decision about procreation.[100] This takes on special relevance with the changes in the timing of counseling. Parents in the past usually received genetic counseling after the birth of a child with genetic disease. Recent advances in genetic technology, such as prenatal diagnosis and carrier detection, enable parents at risk to receive counseling before having children.

Another type of counseling, which might be called family adjustment counseling, becomes an important service in those families with a developmentally defective newborn infant. Some of the same counseling difficulties, paradoxes, and ethical dilemmas can be encountered here as are found in genetic counseling.

ETHICAL IMPLICATIONS FOR NURSING PRACTICE

Many journal articles focused on nursing practice and mental retardation have dealt with ethical dilemmas either indirectly or by implication or not at all.[101-108] Perhaps this lack reflects, among other things, the profound nature of these ethical dilemmas and the difficulties we experience in coming to grips with the emotions that the mentally retarded elicit in us. When we encounter a physically handicapped person, we can experience the encounter as an affront to our own personal integrity in that we realize the fragility of the world that we take for granted. The old adage, "There, but for the grace of God, go I," implies a universal vulnerability in a world over which we do not have absolute control. An encounter with the mentally retarded can be experienced as an affront to the most fundamental core of our own personhood. We react to this affront with a variety of feelings, including thankfulness that we are as we are and guilt that we live in a world of "haves" and "have nots." Another adage comes to mind, "I complained because I had no shoes until I saw the man who had no feet." Old adages have much collected folk wisdom in them and tell us some things about ourselves.

In attempting to cope with such an encounter, commonly experienced feelings of repulsion and disgust not only can prevent us from examining the roots of our reaction, they can also have wide-ranging effects on our definition of the situation and on how or if we deal with the moral claims that the mentally retarded have on us as an individual. Our attitudes also will determine how we think the resources of society should be allocated and how much and what we think the mentally retarded should receive. The concept of *distributive justice* provides us with a moral framework within which to make these decisions.

Obviously, the nurse must first sort out her or his own feelings about and attitudes toward the mentally retarded. Such a sorting out will need to take into account the concept of personhood and where one draws the line, if at all, with regard to the extent of the retardation and the consequences of such action. Questions raised will be: What attitudes do I have toward the mentally retarded? What attitudes should I have and why? Do I tend to stereotype all the mentally retarded and view them as a category rather than as individuals with differences? What moral principles have I used to think through my ethical position vis-à-vis the retarded? What moral claims do the retarded have on me as a professional? What moral claims do they have on society? How do we articulate these claims within the concept of distributive justice?

Parents have reported less than helpful reactions from others, ranging from too much sympathy to denial of any sort of problem to rejection.[109] These and other reactions grounded in negative attitudes toward the mentally retarded can hinder the nurse in performing the basic functions of her or his role, to say nothing of the quality of caring. It can only be assumed that the nurses working directly with the retarded and their families over a period of time have developed a moral position that enables them to provide all of the care required in the situation, while at the same time protecting the rights of these patients. Medicine has been accused of paternalism, but nursing also needs to examine its activities, especially with such patients as the mentally retarded and the mentally ill, to ascertain the extent of the paternalism that we inflict on others. In the sense in which any of us can ever be said to be at home in the world, we are at home not through dominating but through caring for the others in ways that permit both to grow.

More problems may occur for the school nurse, the community nurse, or the nurse in the acute care setting, whose encounters with the retarded have been less frequent and of less intensity. In dealing with the ethical dilemmas of mental retardation, focusing on the rights of the retarded person may be helpful. The official statement of the American Association on Mental Deficiency makes the point that in all activities—designing facilities and organizing services, allocating funds and other resources, participating in the legislative or judicial process, teaching, conducting research, and "most of all, when participating directly in the treatment, training, and habilitation of retarded persons"—the rights of these individuals should serve as the foundation of all else.

For the nurse in the neonatal intensive care unit, the dilemma that she may face over the issue of letting the infant die because he is retarded will call for moral reasoning with regard to the part she can or cannot play in this drama. It can only be hoped that the environment in such a unit will encourage open discussion of these ethical dilemmas in all their complex points.

As the field of genetics further advances, nurses—both practitioners and educators, individually and collectively—along with other health professionals and concerned citizens must become more knowledgeable about the implications of this research. Decisions and research findings in this field affect all of us living now as well as future generations. The need to weigh the potential risks and possible benefits on the future course of human evolution has been addressed often recently. Our deep-rooted concepts of ourselves and our relationship to the universe will be reappraised in this process. This has enormous consequences, not only for the mentally retarded but for all of us. Value judgments inevitably will play an important part in determining the direction society takes on this scientific and ethical issue. One can only wonder if the insights and humility gained from encounters with the mentally retarded will help in this awesome task before us.[110,111] As the largest segment of the health industry, nurses should have some valuable input for this debate. In all of these ethical dilemmas, the moral principles of justice and utility, or the greatest possible balance of good over evil, have a part in our concept of obligations to the mentally retarded, as well as to the rest of us, now and in the future.

REFERENCES

1. Downie RS, Telfer E: *Respect for Persons*. New York: Schocken Books; 1970: p 93.
2. Fletcher JF: Four indicators of humanhood. *Hastings Cent Rep* December 1974.
3. Kant I: *The Fundamental Principles of the Metaphysic of Morals*, Paton HJ (trans). London: Hutchinson's University Library; 1948: pp 90–91.
4. Downie RS, Telfer E: *Respect for Persons*, p 19.
5. English J: Abortion and the concept of a person. *Can J Philos* 5(2), October 1975.
6. Veatch RM: *A Theory of Medical Ethics*. New York: Basic Books; 1981: pp 240–249.
7. Crocker AC, Cushna B: Ethical considerations and attitudes in the field of developmental disorders. In Johnston RB, Magrab PR (eds): *Developmental Disorders: Assessment, Treatment, Education*. Baltimore: University Park Press; 1976: p 496.
8. Friedman PR: *The Rights of Mentally Retarded Persons*. New York: Avon; 1976: pp 57–95.
9. *Ibid.*, pp 97–135.
10. Macklin R, Gaylin W: *Mental Retardation and Sterilization: A Problem of Competency and Paternalism*. New York: Plenum Press; 1981.
11. Annas GJ: Sterilization of the mentally retarded: A decision for the courts. *Hastings Cent Rep* 11:18–19, 1981.
12. Donovan P: Sterlizing the poor and the incompetent. *Hastings Cent Rep* 6:7–8, October 1976.
13. Friedman PR: *Rights of Mentally Retarded*, pp 115–121.
14. Krugman S, Giles JP: Viral hepatitis: New light on an old disease. *JAMA* 212:1019–1021, May 11, 1970.
15. Goldby S: Letter. *Lancet* 7702:749, April 10, 1971.
16. Krugman S: Letter. *Lancet* 7706:966, May 8, 1971.
17. Edsall G: Letter. *Lancet* 7715:95, July 10, 1971.
18. Ramsey P: *The Patient as Person*, New Haven: Yale University Press; 1970: pp 40–58.
19. Milunsky A: *The Prevention of Genetic Diseases and Mental Retardation*. Philadelphia: Saunders; 1975: p 3.
20. Stein Z, Susser M: Public health and mental retardation. In Begab MJ, Richardson SA (eds.): *The Mentally Retarded and Society*. Baltimore: University Park Press; 1974: p 64.
21. *Ibid.*, p 54.
22. *Facts on Mental Retardation*, Washington, DC: National Association for Retarded Children, 1971.
23. Clow CL, Fraser FC, Laberge C, et al: On the application of knowledge to the patient with genetic disease. In Steinberg AG, Bearn AG (eds): *Progress in Medical Genetics*. New York: Grune & Stratton; 1973: vol 9, p 159.

24. McKusick VA: *Mendelian Inheritance in Man*. Baltimore: Johns Hopkins University Press; 1971.

25. Motulsky AG: Population genetics of mental retardation. In Jervis GA (ed): *Expanding Concepts in Mental Retardation*. Springfield, IL: Charles C. Thomas; 1968: p 13.

26. Rothman DJ: *The Discovery of the Asylum: Social Order and Disorder in the New Republic*. Boston: Little, Brown; 1971.

27. Dain N: *Concepts of Insanity in the United States, 1789–1865*. New Brunswick, NJ: Rutgers University Press; 1964.

28. Lazerson M: Educational institutions and mental subnormality: Notes on writing a history. In Begab MJ, Richardson SA (eds): *The Mentally Retarded and Society*. Baltimore: University Park Press; 1974: p 37.

29. Wolfensberger W: The origin and nature of our institutional models. In Kugel RB, Wolfensberger W (eds): *Changing Patterns in Residential Services for the Mentally Retarded*. Washington, DC: President's Committee on Mental Retardation; 1969: pp 59–171.

30. Cremin LA: *The Transformation of the School*. New York: Knopf; 1962.

31. Spring J: *Education and the Rise of the Corporate State*. Boston: Beacon Press; 1972.

32. Lazerson M, Grubb WN: *American Education and Vocationalism, 1870–1970*. New York: Teachers College Press; 1974.

33. Haller M: *Eugenics: Hereditarian Attitudes in American Thought*. New Brunswick, NJ: Rutgers University Press; 1963.

34. Lazerson M, Grubb WN: *American Education*, p 49.

35. White House Conference on Child Health and Protection: *Special Education*. New York: Century; 1931.

36. Blatt B: Some persistently recurring assumptions concerning the mentally subnormal. In Rothstein JH (ed): *Mental Retardation*. New York: Holt, Rinehart, & Winston; 1961: pp 113–125.

37. Begab MJ: Trends and issues. In Begab MJ, Richardson SA: *The Mentally Retarded and Society*. Baltimore: University Park Press; 1974: pp 26–29.

38. Grossman H: *Manual on Terminology and Classification in Mental Retardation*. Washington, DC: American Association for Mental Deficiency; 1973.

39. Anastasi A: *Psychological Testing*. New York: Macmillan; 1968.

40. Edgerton RB: *The Cloak of Competence: Stigma in the Lives of the Mentally Retarded*. Berkeley: University of California Press; 1967.

41. Goffman I: *Stigma: Notes on the Management of Spoiled Identity*. Englewood Cliffs, NJ: Prentice-Hall; 1963.

42. Kleck R, Ono H, Hastorf AH: The effects of physical deviance upon face-to-face interaction. *Hum Relations* 19(4):425–436, 1966.

43. Lippman L: *Attitudes Toward the Handicapped*. Springfield, IL: Charles C. Thomas; 1972.

44. MacMillan DA, Jones RL, Aloia GF: The mentally retarded label: A theoretical analysis and review of research. *Am J Ment Defic* 79:241–261, 1974.

45. Mercer JR: *Labeling the Mentally Retarded*. Berkeley: University of California Press; 1973.

46. Edgerton RB, Sabagh G: From mortification to aggrandizement: Changing self-concepts in the careers of the mentally retarded. *Psychiatry* 25:263–272, 1962.

47. Richardson SA: Reaction to mental subnormality. In Begab MJ, Richardson SA (eds): *The Mentally Retarded and Society*. Baltimore: University Park Press; 1974; p 95.
48. Gottwald H: Public awareness about mental retardation. Research monograph. Arlington, Va., Council for Exceptional Children, 1970.
49. Gottlieb J: Public, peer, and professional attitudes. In Begab MJ, Richardson SA (eds): *The Mentally Retarded and Society*. Baltimore: University Park Press; 1974; p 102.
50. Phelps WR: Attitudes related to the employment of the mentally retarded. *Am J Ment Defic* 69:575–585, 1965.
51. Hollinger CS, Jones RL: Community attitudes toward slow learners and mental retardates. *Ment Retard* 8:19–23, 1970.
52. Gottlieb J, Corman L: Public attitudes toward mentally retarded children. *Am J Ment Defic* 80:72–80, 1975.
53. Johnson GO: Social position of mentally handicapped children in regular grades. *Am J Ment Defic* 55:60–89, 1950.
54. Gottlieb J, Davis JE: Social acceptance of EMRS during overt behavioral interaction. *Am J Ment Defic* 78:141–143, 1973.
55. Iano RP, Ayers D, Heller AB, et al: Sociometric status of retarded children in an integrative program. *Except Child* 40:267–271, 1974.
56. Monroe JD, Howe CE: Effects of integration and social class on the acceptance of retarded adolescents. *Educ Training Ment Retard* 6:20–24, 1971.
57. Meyerowitz JH: Self-derogations in young retardates and special class placement. *Ment Retard* 5:23–26, 1967.
58. Combs RH, Harper JL: Effects of labels on attitudes of educators toward handicapped children. *Except Child* 33:399–403, 1967.
59. Alper S, Retish PM: A comparative study of the effects of student teaching in the attitudes of students in special education, elementary education, and secondary education. *Training School Bull* 69:70–77, 1972.
60. Shotel JR, Iano RP, McGettigan JF: Teacher attitude associated with the integration of handicapped children. *Except Child* 38:677–683, 1972.
61. Parsons T: The school class as a social system. *Harvard Educ Rev* 29:297–315, 1959.
62. Turner R: Sponsored and contest mobility and the school system. *Am Soc Rev* 25:855–867, 1960.
63. Cicourel A, Kitsuse J: *The Educational Decisionmakers*. New York: Bobbs-Merrill; 1963.
64. Jencks C: *Inequality: A Reassessment of the Effect of Family and Schooling in America*. New York: Basic Books; 1972.
65. Rosenthal R, Jacobson L: *Pygmalion in the Classroom: Teacher Expectation and Pupil's Intellectual Development*. New York: Holt, Rinehart, Winston; 1968.
66. Lapp ER: A study of the social adjustment of slow-learning children who were assigned part-time to regular classes. *Am J Ment Defic* 62:254–262, 1959.
67. Stone AA: *Mental Health and Law: A System in Transition*. HEW, National Institute of Mental Health, 1975; pp 119–140.
68. Brakel S, Rock R: *The Mentally Disabled and the Law*. Chicago: University of Chicago Press; 1971: pp 98–102.

69. Ennis B, Friedman PR: *Legal Rights of the Mentally Handicapped*. New York: Practising Law Institute; 1973: pp 15–101.
70. Murdock CW: Civil rights of the mentally retarded: Some critical issues. *Notre Dame Lawyer* 48:133–188, 1972.
71. *The Decisive Decade*. Washington, DC: The President's Committee on Mental Retardation; 1970.
72. *Wyatt v Stickney*, 325 F Supp 781 M.D. (AL, 1971).
73. *Who Should Survive?* film. Joseph P. Kennedy, Jr. Foundation for the International Symposium on Human Rights, Retardation and Research, Washington, DC, 1971.
74. Brakel S, Rock R: *Mentally Disabled*.
75. *Townsend v Treadway*, Civil No. 6500, M.D., (TN, 1972).
76. DeLaCruz F, Laveck FD: *Human Sexuality and the Mentally Retarded*. New York: Brunner/Mazel; 1973.
77. Birnbaum M: The right to treatment. *Am Bar Assoc J* 46:499–503, 1960.
78. *Rouse v Cameron*, 373 F2d 451 (DC Cir 1966).
79. *Covington v Harris*, 419 F2d 617 (DC Cir 1969).
80. *Wyatt v Stickney*, Civil No. 3195–N, M.D. (AL 1972).
81. *Annual Report*. Washington, DC, The President's Committee on Mental Retardation; 1969.
82. Murdock CW: Civil rights, p 171.
83. *Roe v Wade*, 410 US 113 (1973).
84. President's Commission for the Study of Ethical Problems in Medicine and Biomedical and Behavioral Research: *Genetic Screening*. Government Printing Office, 1983.
85. Childs B: Genetic screening. In Roman HL (ed): *Annual Review of Genetics*. Palo Alto, CA: Annual Reviews; 1975: vol 9, pp 67–89.
86. Lappé M: *Genetic Politics: The Limits of Biological Control*. New York: Simon & Schuster; 1979: pp 26–27.
87. Reilly R: *Genetics, Law and Social Policy*. Cambridge, MA: Harvard University Press; 1977: p 44.
88. Levy HL: Genetic screening. In Harris H, Hirschhorn, K (eds): *Advances in Human Genetics*. New York: Plenum Press; 1973: vol 4, p 3.
89. Bessman SP, Swazey JP: Phenylketonuria: A study of biomedical legislation. In Mendelsohn E, Swazey JP, Jarvis L (eds): *Human Aspects of Biomedical Innovation*. Cambridge, MA: Harvard University Press; 1971: pp 49–76.
90. Reilly P: State supported mass genetic screening programs. In A Milunsky A, Annas GJ (eds): *Genetics and the Law*. New York: Plenum Press; 1976: p 160.
91. *Ibid.*, p 161.
92. Levy HL, Genetic screening, pp 32–34.
93. Reilly P; *Genetics, Law and Social Policy*, p 65.
94. The National Sickle Cell Anemia, Cooley's Anemia, Tay-Sachs and Genetic Diseases Act, Pub L No. 92–278, 90 Stat, tit IV, § 401; 1976.
95. Reilly PR: The role of law in the prevention of genetic disease. In Milunsky A (ed): *The Prevention of Genetic Diseases and Mental Retardation*. Philadelphia: Saunders; 1975: pp 428–429.
96. *Ibid.*, pp 436–437.

97. Milunsky A: Genetic counseling: principles and practice. In Milunsky A (ed): *The Prevention of Genetic Diseases and Mental Retardation.* Philadelphia: Saunders; 1975: pp 64–65.
98. World Health Organization Expert Committee: *Genetic Counseling.* WHO Tech Rep 416:1, 1969.
99. Sorenson JR: Counselors: Self portrait. *Genetic Counseling* 1:31, 1973.
100. Capron AM: Informed decision-making in genetic counseling. *Indiana Law J* 48;581, 1973.
101. Gibson BS, Reed JC: Training nurses in mental retardation. *Ment Retard* 12(6):19–22, 1974.
102. Smiley CW: Sterilization and therapeutic abortion counseling for the mentally retarded. *J Psychiatr Nurs* 12:24–26, May/June 1974.
103. Mahoney JA: Viewpoints on attitudes and actions towards handicapped children. *J Pract Nurs* 24: 40–41, April 1974.
104. Symposium on the child with developmental disabilities. *Nurs Clin North Am* June 1975.
105. Haynes M: Teaching mental retardation nursing. *Am J Nurs* 75:626–628, April 1975.
106. Hume PJ: Perspectives in nursing the mentally handicapped. *World MR Nurs* June 1975, pp 6–7
107. Branson HK: The nurse's role in behavior modification. *Nurs Care* 8:21–23, December 1975.
108. Thurman RL, Smowe RJ: The nurse practitioner and institutional facilities for the mentally retarded: Are they compatible? *J Psychiatr Nurs* 14:7–10, May 1976.
109. Horoshak I: Where hope for mental retardees grows brighter: Eunice Kennedy Shriver Center for Mental Retardation. *RN* 39:39–43, June 1976.
110. Hannam C: *Parents and Mentally Handicapped Children.* Baltimore: Penguin Books; 1975: p 48.
111. Mayeroff M: *On Caring.* New York: Harper & Row; 1971.

CHAPTER 12

Public Policy and Health Care Delivery

Individually and collectively nurses are involved in development and implementation of policy in institutions and communities in the public and private sectors. Examples of this involvement range from policies that determine allocation of nursing care and expertise in hospitals and nursing homes to legislative actions related to advance treatment decisions and the allocation of health care resources to and within health care delivery systems. Generally, policy refers to a course of action or inaction selected from among alternatives in the context of given conditions to guide present and future decisions and implementation of those decisions. The American Nurses' Association (ANA) document *Nursing: A Social Policy Statement* (1980) is one example within the nursing profession.

Public policy consists of a course of action chosen by government.[1] The principles guiding such choices are or should be the concern of everyone in society. Health policy issues and ethics intersect in such considerations as the allocation of health care and nursing expertise to individuals, groups and communities at local, state, national, and international levels.

All health policy issues involve ethical-value dimensions that are often not considered explicitly in debate that focuses on economic and political factors. Yet, it is such ethical values as adequate access to health care and respect for individual autonomy that should guide policy decisions. Values may be considered to be a set of beliefs and attitudes for which logical reasons can be given. Values are significant as they influence our perceptions of situations, guide our actions, and have consequences. Not all values are ethical or moral values. There are also political, economic, aesthetic, and other types of values that enter into policy decisions.

Arguments and decisions about health policy are ultimately based on underlying assumptions about what is valued in society and where health is placed on the list of societal priorities. This is significant to nurses as health care providers and to consumers of health care and nursing care, for it means that finite resources must be allocated among such competing societal interests as education, housing, defense, and welfare broadly and more narrowly within health care. Curative and preventive care, education of health workers, and research represent competing interests and claims on health dollars.

Fuchs, an economist, points out in his now classic book *Who Should Live?* that resources are scarce, resources have alternative uses, and individuals have different wants and attach different levels of importance to satisfying these wants.[2] Notice that Fuchs talks about wants, not needs. Needs could be used as one basis for distribution of benefits and burdens in a just fashion in health care delivery. The three factors mentioned by Fuchs indicate that choices must be made at personal and social levels in order to resolve issues such as the fairest distribution of resources to health care: who is to choose for communities and nations, how priorities will be set, and how needs and interests of individuals and society will be reconciled in policy development. These and numerous other issues reflect value conflicts in our pluralistic society, such as individual freedom of choice and avoiding harm to others in the community.

Two of the overall purposes of government, as found in the Preamble to the US Constitution, are promoting the general welfare and establishing justice. Public policy is developed within this constitutional framework to meet these goals. According to Strickland, the policy-making process consists of deciding on goals for the public good and delineating and activating strategies for achieving these goals. This process requires agreement on both means and ends among those who have effective control over resources, such as money, personnel, and facilities.[3] A national health policy per se does not exist if one considers the following four aspects essential to policy: clear statement of purpose, working consensus to achieve the purpose, agreement on both means and ends, and continuing fiscal support of composite programs.[4] Much American medical care is still focused primarily on cure of disease and the use of increasingly sophisticated high tech procedures. Preventive activities are encouraged, yet most insurance still provides coverage only for hospital care and physicians' services in the hospital. Relatively few people have insurance coverage for preventive or ambulatory care while an increasing number of individuals are uninsured or underinsured for medical care. We know that medical care is a major (but not the only) factor contributing to health. Medical care does not equal health care.

Even if we do not have a national health policy in the United States, the federal budget of the executive branch and health legislation for authorizing particular appropriations reflect implicit values about obligations in and to health care. They provide a foundation for policy making as they reflect the place of health and health care politically, economically, and ethically in the overall societal picture. They impact the allocation of medical resources, health personnel, and the provision of personal, community, and environmental health services at primary, secondary, and tertiary levels. In other words, they have consequences for the lives and well-being of people.

HISTORICAL AND LEGISLATIVE BACKGROUND

Historical and legislative aspects discussed here demonstrate the ways that values and value conflicts related to health have been part of our history as a country from its early beginnings. Health care has moved into an increasingly prominent place on the national public policy agenda as costs have escalated and various interventions, voluntary and mandated, have been used unsuccessfully in attempts to contain these costs. The increasing numbers of people who are uninsured or underinsured and lack adequate access to health care have also focused public concern on health and health care. Government's commitment to health care on the public policy agenda has changed over time and can be traced historically in legislation and funds actually appropriated to implement the legislation. These commitments have affected nursing education, nursing research, and the delivery of nursing care directly and indirectly.

Hints of a national health policy can be identified from the time of establishment of the Colonies. Early health measures passed by the Colonies in the late 1600s had to do with quarantine for communicable disease control. Further quarantine laws were passed by individual states to control yellow fever. In the 1790s, the actual occurrence and continuing threat of yellow fever and its effect on the economy forced the new Congress to pass legislation giving the President power to state the conditions of quarantine. At the time, the debate focused primarily on state versus federal authority rather than health matters per se. In 1813, Congress went further in committing the federal government to more involvement with preservation of the health of citizens; a vaccination law was passed to make effective cowpox vaccine available to anyone requesting it free of charge. This law was repealed after the wrong vaccine was sent to the state of North Carolina, with disastrous results. But a precedent was set for involvement of the federal government in the health of individual citizens.[5]

In the late 1800s, the American Medical Association (AMA) made a definite distinction between public health and private, individual health. "State medicine" was to benefit communities by dealing with such communicable diseases as smallpox, which could only be controlled through public efforts. Even at that time there were problems in this public-or-private distinction, which rapidly became blurred. Conflict began to develop between private groups, such as the AMA, and the government over governmental involvement in health. Another yellow fever epidemic in the 1870s influenced the authorization of a National Board by the federal government. The Board's duties were rather vague. But in the four years of its existence, it did authorize funds for biomedical research.[6]

Problems continued with the quarantine law and the authority to enforce it. Eventually, authority was given to the Marine Hospital Service, which became the United States Public Health Service in 1912. The Public Health Service was authorized to do epidemiological research in order to control and prevent disease. Preventive medicine and the health of the public were still the bases of the general philosophy for government in health matters. Curative medicine and the health of individuals were considered to be primarily private concerns.[7]

European social and health insurance schemes began to receive attention in the United States in the early 1900s. The climate of economic reform in the United States, demands for better working conditions, emergence of labor unions, and passage of the National Health Insurance Act in Britain (1911) stimulated this interest. In the United States, the American Section of the International Association for Labor Legislation promoted the health insurance cause by calling for insurance against accidents, sickness, old age, and unemployment, further indication that health concerns require personal *and* collective action. Government recognition of social and health needs was reflected in presidential messages, beginning early in the twentieth century. Federally sponsored health insurance was at least mentioned in many of the presidential messages but was not activated through legislation. Early in the twentieth century, the AMA was *not* opposed to some form of health insurance. This lack of opposition soon ended.[8]

The Great Depression and the passage of the Social Security Act in 1935 saw further federal concern over health, even though the Social Security Board had no charge directly related to health insurance when the Act was passed in its final form. In 1939, Senator Robert F. Wagner introduced an amendment to the social security law called the National Health Act of 1939. This was followed in the early 1940s by several attempts to pass the Murray–Wagner–Dingell Bill, which would have created a system of federal compulsory health insurance and federal support of medical education. This proposal was strongly opposed by the private side of medical care, the AMA, and never came to a vote. However, the AMA did support the Hill–Burton Bill later, in 1946. This provided grants-in-aid to hospitals via the states for hospital construction. This program was steadily extended in the form of grants for such projects as research on hospital utilization, construction of nursing homes and other facilities, and hospital modernization projects.[9] This was part of an overall effort to improve services to citizens. This legislation accurately demonstrates the philosophy of "sick care" in public policy making, rather than health care.

Legislative forerunners to Medicare began to appear in the late 1950s and early 1960s in the Forand Bill and the Kerr–Mills Bill, which became law in 1960. The Forand Bill provided hospital and medical care for the elderly through Social Security. The Kerr–Mills Bill did not use the social security mechanism for financing but provided federal aid to the states for payments for medical care of the "medically indigent" elderly.[10] Before Medicare and Medicaid (Social Security Amendments of 1965) were finally passed, the AMA did introduce its own proposal, Eldercare, which also excluded the social security financing mechanism. Medicare and Medicaid make no provisions for change in the actual structure of health care delivery.

Medicaid provides grants to states for medical assistance programs. Matching federal grants are made available to the states, at state option, for a medical assistance program for such groups as recipients of federally aided public assistance, recipients of supplemental security income benefits, the medically indigent in comparable groups (families with dependent children as defined for public assistance purposes, the aged, the blind, and the disabled), and other indigent children. Services include in-hospital services, out-patient hospital services, other laboratory and x-ray services, skilled nursing home services, physicians' services, screening programs for children, and family planning services. Medicaid is usually administered through the Department of Public Welfare, Social Services, or Human Services at the discretion of the individual states.[11]

A look at the Social Security Act Titles passed through the past five decades demonstrates increasing involvement of the federal government in efforts to make health and medical care benefits available to an ever-increasing number of groups, such as the elderly, the disabled, and children. A similar trend can be seen in the Public Health Service Act of 1944. This Act legislated particular activities related to research and investigation of both physical and mental health problems, federal–state cooperation in prevention and control of communicable disease, and medical care to specified groups, such as merchant seamen and federal employees. Under this Act, the National Cancer Institute was established, as were Regional Medical Programs (Heart Disease, Cancer, and Stroke Amendments of 1965) and Health Manpower legislation (1960), providing grants for training in public health and nursing.[12]

The Comprehensive Health Planning Amendments were passed in 1966. One purpose of this legislation was to encourage comprehensive health planning through establishment of state-and area-wide comprehensive health planning including providers and consumers. They did not specifically attempt to change the delivery of health care in any major way. The Health Maintenance Organization Act of 1973 provided financial assistance for the development of health maintenance organizations, which include prepaid group medical practice. This is the first deliberate legislative effort at the federal level to reorganize the delivery of health care.[13]

The 1972 Social Security Amendments are of particular note, as they made important changes in the Social Security Act, including Medicare and Medicaid. These Amendments also established Performance Standards Review Organizations (PSROs) directed to problems of control of cost, quality, and medical necessity of services. PSROs were established in states for review of professional activities of physicians and other providers. Another provision was for treatment of chronic renal disease under Medicare with reimbursement provided for hemodialysis or renal transplantation.[14]

PL 93–641, the National Health Planning and Resource Development Act of 1974, combined many of the activities of the Hill–Burton Bill, Regional Medical Programs, and Comprehensive Health Planning into one single network of authority with Health Systems Agencies (HSAs) in designated health service areas. Federal funding, coming into a geographic area for planning and development of health services, went through agencies composed of providers and a majority of consumers on the HSA board or executive committee.[15]

Appropriation of increasing amounts of funding for medical research and development of the National Institutes of Health during the past few decades represented a significant level of governmental support for these activities. The amount of funding is now being cut drastically, reflecting a national change in support for health care activities. At the same time, states are being required to deal with decreased federal funding levels and the change from categorical grants to block grants, raising further issues of access and equity.

Further development of federal commitment to the support of health personnel development occurred in the 1960s and 1970s. Funding in various forms was appropriated for training of physicians, dentists, pharmacists, nurses, podiatrists, and allied health professionals. Construction grants, improvement grants, student loan funds, scholarships, and capitation grants were provided to educational and health institutions. The Comprehensive Health Manpower Training Act of 1971 provided for a new program of grants, contracts, and health manpower education initiative awards for the purpose of "improving the distribution, supply, quality, utilization, and efficiency of health personnel and the health services delivery system."[16] This level of support has decreased.

This very brief overview of legislative patterns related to health matters reflects value judgments and critical choices made over the years in allocation of finite resources, from control of communicable disease to development of medical research, health manpower, financing mechanisms for medical and health care, and efforts to alter health care delivery structures. Federal concerns about the health of citizens is also reflected in other kinds of legislation not discussed here, such as legislation for regulation of the pharmaceutical industry, and health and safety in the work place.

HEALTH CARE POLICY—THE PAST TWO DECADES

Radical changes surrounding and influencing health care policy occurred in the 1970s and 1980s. Rapidly rising health care costs that now consume more than 11.5 percent of the Gross National Product (GNP) and unsuccessful attempts to deal with them have had the greatest role in shaping today's health care system. Managed care plans combining insurance and provider functions, horizontal integration of health care facilities into large multi-institutional organizations, expansion of hospitals into ambulatory surgery, home care, substance abuse clinics, and other services, implementation of Medicare's Diagnostic Related Groups (DRG) system, and adoption of a resource-based relative-value scale (RBVS) for Medicare payments to physicians represent extraordinary changes in delivery of health care in the United States. All of these efforts demonstrate a policy priority of trying to deal with escalating costs ". . . almost to the exclusion of any other policy objectives."[17] This priority and the efforts to put it into operation have obscured the impact that these changes have had on traditional ethical values in medicine and health care such as professional autonomy, patient autonomy, advocacy for patients, and the fullest possible access to health care.[18] Another important aspect of these changes and efforts to deal with them effectively is the nursing shortage in many parts of the country because of a greater demand for nursing expertise. These profound changes in the delivery of health care and the challenge to traditional values point more clearly than ever to the interface of ethics and politics as society deals with issues such as the allocation and rationing of resources in health care. What are some of the dimensions of ethically responsible health and public policy?

ETHICAL DIMENSIONS OF PUBLIC POLICY

> *The realm of politics is a twilight zone*
> *where ethical and technical issues meet.*
> Reinhold Niebuhr

Social scientists Kelman and Warwick, writing on the ethics of social intervention in the 1970s, present a framework that is significant to public policy development and implementation. They see social intervention on a continuum from national policy to policy making in organizations and experimentation with human subjects. Social intervention is regarded as any planned or unplanned action that changes characteristics of an individual or the pattern of relationships among individuals.[19] In this discussion, the focus is on the latter concept as we consider issues in social and political arenas related to health care policy.

Warwick and Kelman discuss four areas of intervention that raise ethical concerns that should be addressed *before* policies are developed and implemented in order to develop more ethically responsible and responsive policy. This framework can also be used to identify and evaluate ethical aspects of existing policies in organizations and in public policy. The four areas are:[20]

1. The choice of policy goals that maximize or minimize specific values, as in prospective reimbursement systems that have cost containment as a major purpose and maximize economic values and minimize human values, such as respect for individual autonomy and access for all to needed health care;
2. The definition of the target of change, that is, who or what is supposed to change—clients, providers, organizations—and how are they involved in the process of policy development or revision?
3. The means chosen to develop and implement policy, ranging from coercive to facilitative means in which both respect for individual autonomy and the welfare of society are taken seriously;
4. Assessment of direct and indirect consequences of a proposed policy to the greatest extent possible, such as looking at economic and emotional and psychological costs (a distributive justice concern) to all affected directly and indirectly by the policy, such as individual clients, families, caregivers, and communities.

One example might be a major effort by government to focus policies on preventive health activities in the areas of personal and environmental health. Such policy efforts would maximize the value of the greatest good for the greatest number, a utilitarian view. At the same time, this might have negative effects on the values of equity and justice for the very sick elderly. In this example, the choice for targets of change might be individual life styles and modifying carcinogenic elements in the environment. Methods of inducing change might impinge on values of individual freedom and autonomy or on the freedom of industry to maximize profits. Conflict might occur between groups educating for life-style changes and those working for healthier air and water as they compete for finite resources. Finally, one has to assess the risks and benefits of various consequences of proposed policy changes on traditional values such as advocacy for individual patients. If decision makers opt for expenditure of public funds on educating for life-style changes, there is the potential for developing the "victim blaming" syndrome. What, if any, values such as personal freeedom are we willing or unwilling to give up or have modified in the interests of a healthier society?

A key issue in examining goals of intervention and means for implementing change is the extent to which affected population groups have their values and interests represented in the process, such as various socioeconomic groups, men, women, children, the employed, the unemployed, the healthy, the sick, providers, and consumers. How much control do the affected groups and individuals have in the process of change? Whose interests are being served by the proposed intervention, the providers of a community health program or the target population? Is the power of one group strengthened at the expense of another? All of these concerns should be considered in any process of social intervention. They often are not, because of the difficulty in discerning which values should predominate and the difficulty of predicting consequences of particular actions on any selected value, such as the individual's freedom of choice or the overall welfare of society.[21]

The concerns of moral philosophy about the "right" and the "good" are not usually considered explicitly in developing public policy. Jonsen, a bioethicist, and Butler, a professor of health policy, suggest some specific ways that ethical dimensions can be added to policy debate. In proposing that ethical considerations be part of public policy debate, there are several problems that make this dialogue difficult[22]:

1. exploring the ethics of a policy proposal does not provide ready-made answers for which action is right in a given situation;
2. the ethics has its own special language;
3. there is a common conception that ethics has to do primarily with personal behavior;
4. policy makers have constituencies with loyalties and interests, which ethicists do not; and
5. policy makers use the technical expertise of others in making decisions but feel that in ethics and moral judgments one is one's own expert.

Yet both ethicists and policy makers are concerned about what is "good" for society and for individual members of that society. Some concepts of politics speak to politics as a branch of ethics concerned with ethical relations and duties of governments and other social organizations. This notion negates the idea that ethics is *solely* a personal matter. Furthermore, politics deals with conflicting needs and interest, as does applied ethics.

Jonsen and Butler see "public ethics" as a subset of social ethics. "Public ethics" deals with public, that is, governmental decisions about matters of public concern, such as a safe and adequate water supply and equitable access to health care; deals with pressing issues that must be decided, such as expenditure of public funds; and usually does not have the goal of creating significant structural change in society but involves relatively minor modifications in social or economic arrangements. The three tasks of "public ethics" are: (1) to articulate the moral principles most relevant to the policy problem under consideration, such as justice, equity, and respect for persons; (2) to examine proposed policy choices in view of identified relevant moral principals; and (3) to rank in order the moral options for a particular policy choice. This is rather like a "moral balance sheet" in terms of which social or economic arrangements enhance one moral principle and not another.[23]

In looking at the development of a national health insurance system, Jonsen and Butler considered two moral principles: distributive justice (fair distribution of harms and benefits in society according to standards of equity, desert, need, or contract) and respect for individuals (implies equal treatment for each person who has sets of liberties, rights, and obligations). What follows is one example of how a discussion might evolve between a congressman and an ethicist. In bringing the concept of distributive justice into the debate about national health insurance, many questions would be raised. Questions and concerns would include the distribution of burdens and benefits to particular groups in society, whether or not equality is a criterion for distribution, the justification of unequal distribution according to merit or ability, and whether there is an "objective" way to determine a "fair" distribution in terms of the most medically needy.[24]

In clarifying policy options, one must, for example, consider the impact of deductibles and coinsurance on the poor, who may be particularly discouraged by them from seeking medical care. If relatively small deductibles are paid by patients, the money "saved" by government could be used for the seriously or chronically ill who must be institutionalized for care. However, wouldn't it be more just to still provide "free" care for the very poor? This might be considered unfair for those who do pay the deductible, because there would be less money "saved" to be used for the more expensive care. The ethicist might then show that the criterion of medical need takes preference over the criterion of equality, such as the need arising from poverty, which does influence negatively the distribution patterns of illness and disease. In the Rawlsian tradition, one might claim that it is not "unfair" to improve the position of the least advantaged in society. In view of fiscal constraints, some rationing of care is thought by some to be necessary. It might be more just to have a plan based on balancing the respective needs of the very sick, the very poor, and the uninsured. Deductibles would vary with income, so that the very poor would pay almost nothing. One can consider "equity" factors in various proposals in addition to economic evaluation of cost effectiveness, administrative implications, and changes in health care delivery patterns.[25] Such considerations would add an ethical dimension to health policy debate and decisions, as in the state of Oregon, where public forums were held to discuss ethical principles that should inform state legislation about health care.

Further considerations that should inform public policy debate about health care were developed in the report of the President's Commission for the Study of Ethical Problems in Medicine and Biomedical and Behavioral Research (1983) on access to health care and in the proposals made by Daniel Callahan in his book entitled *What Kind of Life: The Limits of Medical Progress* (1989). The President's Commission concluded that society has an ethical obligation to ensure equitable access to health care for all. This ethical obligation rests on the special importance of health care to relief of suffering, prevention of premature death, restoration of functioning, increasing opportunity, provision of information about individual health status, and showing evidence of mutual empathy and compassion.[26] Additional conclusions related to balancing societal and individual obligations to share fairly the costs of health care; ensuring that all citizens are able to secure an adequate level of care without excessive burdens; that the ultimate responsibility for ensuring that societal obligations are met rests with the federal government; and that while efforts to contain health care costs are important, they should not focus on limiting access to the most vulnerable population groups in our society.[27] Various public and private groups and organizations, including business and industry, continue to struggle with what constitutes an adequate level of care for all.

Callahan's proposals point to the fact that health is not an end in and of itself.[28] He asserts that health can only have meaning in the context of the overall welfare of our society, that is, the welfare of our social, educational, economic, and cultural institutions. He proposes a different vision of medical progress that gives the highest priority to caring for those who cannot be cured for a variety of reasons such as scientific, physiological, or economic realities. No one should be abandoned and should always be treated with compassion as a member of the human community. The next priority would focus on the principles and practices of public health and primary care as they are most conducive to the common good at the least cost. Examples include good nutrition, disease prevention, immunizations, antibiotics, primary care, and emergency medicine. Last, society should pursue the advanced forms of high-technology medicine that tend to benefit fewer individuals at comparatively high costs. Organ transplants and advanced intensive care services are examples. These would be priorities to guide policy, and they represent a radical shift from today's priorities of cure at almost any financial, emotional, or psychological costs.

Allocation of health care resources in relation to other societal institutions and needs requires some degree of societal consensus about our health goals. Callahan raises the question of whether the search for unlimited medical progress may not lead to the impoverishment of the rest of our lives. He claims that we have drifted along for years ". . . creating a health care system that not only costs too much for what it delivers, but fails also to deliver what it could for millions of people . . . [and] has led us to spend too much on health in comparison with other social needs, too much on the old in comparison with the young, too much on the acutely ill in comparison with the chronically ill, too much on curing in comparison with caring. . . and too much on extending the length of life rather than enhancing the quality of life."[29] Any serious health policy debates must take account of the work of the President's Commission and Callahan's proposals in order to represent policy recommendations that are more than simply attempts to deal with economic and cost considerations with little regard for the values driving policy decisions.

In summary, some ways of incorporating ethical aspects and arguments in health policy development have been discussed. The work of the President's Commission and Callahan suggest further ethical content focused on obligations for policy decisions affecting the health and welfare of individuals and of our society. The ideas presented here can and should also be used to inform ethically responsible institutional policies.

FURTHER THOUGHTS FOR NURSING

The nurse collaborates with members of the health professions and other citizens in promoting community and national efforts to meet the health needs of the public.

ANA Code for Nurses, 1985

Accountability to the patient or client and collaboration with other health professionals for purposes of ensuring access to needed health and nursing care require a reasoned decision-making process. One of the principles nurses, both individually and collectively, can use in looking at the interface of ethics and politics in policy development and assessment is distributive justice, which considers the distribution of burdens and benefits in society. Nurses and others must take this into account in attempting to meet the health and nursing needs of individuals, families, and communities and to ensure the survival of organizations to deliver health services.

Nurses are becoming more knowledgeable and involved in public policy development and assessment.[30-33] Nursing values such as belief in individual rights to health care and respect for human dignity provide a foundation for nursing involvement in health care policy development.[34]

Using medical and nursing needs as a basis for distribution of benefits of health care and for a perspective on rights to and obligations in health care, needs might be considered as a spectrum extending from needs that arise in the individual, such as those created by life-threatening illness, through needs for prevention of disease, to needs that arise in the physical environment—the life support system of all of us. These needs include safe water, safe food supplies, safe working conditions, and clean air. All of these needs that are required to carry out reasonable life plans for each of us and for the welfare of society are related to physical, mental, and spiritual health. They compete with other social needs and interests, such as public education, for limited societal resources. Nurses can and are taking leadership to articulate such needs in policy making in institutional and governmental arenas.

There are several major decisions that individual nurses, groups of nurses, and professional nursing organizations can make, related to: (1) the types of health and health-related organizations and at what level (local, state, national, or international) they will participate; (2) the type of participation—that is, financial support for groups working on goals that one supports, observer, observer-participant, or active participant; and, finally (3) whether or not nursing will take a stronger initiative in developing ethically responsible and responsive health policy. Specific actions in the ethical domain related to policy assessment and development include: (1) questioning the goals of proposed policies or changes in existing policies; (2) clearly identifying the targets of change and their participation in policy assessment and development processes; (3) identifying the underlying ethical assumptions of policies; (4) discussing means proposed to implement policy changes; (5) assessing the short- and long-term consequences of policy proposals or changes to the greatest degree possible; and (6) identifying the moral principles and values that are at stake in policy changes. Taking such actions in health policy development and assessment processes can lead to different policy decisions from those that occur without such reflection and discussion. Acting in the spirit of "preventive ethics" integrated with sensitivity to political power considerations will not lead automatically to one ethically acceptable decision or policy. Such analysis will rule out certain policy proposals that cannot be justified ethically, such as those that completely ignore the impact of a proposed policy on respect for individual autonomy or equity in access to health care for the most vulnerable.[35] It is a moral imperative that the impact of health policy development and assessment on those such as the sickest individuals, the dying, pregnant women and children, ethnic minorities, and the elderly poor always be taken seriously.

Nurses, and particularly nurse executives, can and should become more knowledgeable about the interaction of social, ethical, legal, economic, and political aspects in institutional and public policy decisions

They can seek to influence these decisions individually and collectively through professional organizations or other community groups in both public and private sectors. Expertise is one form of power, and choosing to do nothing is a choice that has consequences for nursing and its clients. Making ethically responsible decisions for action requires a re-examination of values underlying the rhetoric of nursing and the behavior of nursing and nurses in patient, colleague, organizational, and community relationships. For example, what does the claim that the nurse is a patient advocate imply in terms of institutional policy making and development of adequate systems of nursing care, particularly in instances of nursing shortages?

The tasks involved in development of ethically responsible policy for health service organizations and government are difficult and complex. They require the thinking and action of nurses and others in health care systems who affect and are affected by delivery of nursing care. If an underlying value and practice is to please everyone, that value will be reflected in behavior rather than the value of providing leadership to meet patients' and society's needs for nursing and health *care*. This poses a tremendous challenge to nursing education policy and to *all* institutions that provide nursing services in acute care, long-term care, psychiatric care, home care, prisons, schools, and the workplace.

Ethical concerns in health policy development and assessment are explicitly articulated by the nursing profession in practice, education, and research and can be more so. As a society, we are challenged to develop policies reflective of ethical principles and values. These are essential considerations in decisions about the allocation of finite resources at all levels of government and in health service organizations. While such deliberations are not easy in today's competitive and turbulent health care systems, such reflection and action are vital to meeting nursing's social mandate. Health policy affects all of us as individuals and as members of society and the environments in which we live and work.

REFERENCES

1. Kalisch BJ, Kalisch PA: *Politics of Nursing*. Philadelphia: Lippincott; 1982: p 61.
2. Fuchs VR: *Who Shall Live?* New York: Basic Books; 1974: p 4.
3. Strickland SP: *Politics, Science, and Dread Disease*, Cambridge, MA: Harvard University; 1972: pp x–xi.
4. *Ibid.*, p 255.
5. Chapman CB, Talmadge JM: The evolution of the right to health concept in United States. *Pharos* 34:31–33, January 1971.
6. *Ibid.*, p 35.
7. *Ibid.*, pp 35–36.

8. *Ibid.*, pp 40–42.
9. Stevens R: *American Medicine and the Public Interest.* New Haven: Yale University Press 1971: p 510.
10. Wilson FA, Neuhauser D: *Health Services in the United States*, ed 2. Cambridge, MA: Ballinger; 1982: 170.
11. *Ibid.*, pp 172–179.
12. *Ibid.*, pp 187–189.
13. *Ibid.*, pp 208–210.
14. *Ibid.*, pp 176–180.
15. Novello DJ: The National Health Planning and Resources Development Act. *Nurs Outlook* 24:354–358, June 1976.
16. Wilson FA, Neuhauser D: *Health Services*, pp 203–204.
17. Priester R: Health-care values buried by cost-control emphasis. *Minnesota*, 7:1, January 30, 1990.
18. The Center for Biomedical Ethics: *Rethinking Medical Morality: The Ethical Implications of Changes in Health Care Organization, Delivery, and Financing.* Minneapolis: University of Minnesota; 1989.
19. Warwick DP, Kelman HC: Ethical issues in social intervention. In Bennis WG, Benne KD, Chin R, et al (eds.), ed. 3. New York: Holt, Rinehart, & Winston; 1976: p 470.
20. *Ibid.*, p 471.
21. *Ibid.*, p 476.
22. Jonsen AR, Butler LH: Public ethics and policy making. *Hastings Cent Rep* 5:20–21, August 1975.
23. *Ibid.*, pp 23–24.
24. *Ibid.*, p 28.
25. *Ibid.*, pp 28–29.
26. President's Commission for the Study of Ethical Problems in Medicine and Biomedical and Behavioral Research: *Securing Access to Health Care*, Report. Government Printing Office, 1983: vol 1, p 4.
27. *Ibid.*, pp 4–6.
28. Callahan D: *What Kind of Life?: The Limits of Medical Progress.* New York: Simon & Schuster; 1989.
29. Callahan D: Modernizing mortality: medical progress and the good society. *Hastings Cent Rep*, 20:28–30, January/February 1990.
30. Rowell PA, Knauss PJ: The legislative task force: A method to increase nurses' political involvement. *Nurs Outlook* 29:715–716, December 1981.
31. Harrington C: Quality, access and costs: Public policy and home health care. *Nurs Outlook* 36:164–166, July/August 1988.
32. Miramontes H: Needed: Effective national policy on AIDS/HIV infection. *Nurs Outlook* 36:262–263, 296, November/December 1988.
33. Oda D: The imperative of a national strategy for children: Is there a political will? *Nurs Outlook* 37:206–208, September/October 1989.
34. Davis GC: Nursing values and health care policy. *Nurs Outlook* 36:289–292, November-December 1988.
35. Aroskar MA: The interface of ethics and politics in nursing. *Nurs Outlook* 35:268–272, November-December 1987.

CHAPTER 13

Ethical Dilemmas for Discussion

*Good decision making . . . seems to require human sensitivity, illuminating and useful principles, access to pertinent information, methods weighting and balancing options—reason and feeling, private meditation and public discussion, good sense and good sensibilities.**

D. Callahan

Hypothetical ethical dilemmas for nurses and other health workers are presented in this chapter. There are two case studies for each of Chapters 6 through 12. Each of the related chapters contains content helpful for consideration in making ethical decisions in dilemmas. The reader may wish to review Chapters 2, 3, and 4 before working with the case studies. In each of these situations, the individual or group is seeking the best solution for a given situation where, for example, there is a conflict of duties and obligations, a line is drawn or needs to be drawn, or a moral principle is being or has been violated.

A Decision-making Process

In order to think systematically about the ethical dilemmas in the case studies, one should consider some basic elements. The first element to be considered is the available data base, which includes individuals involved and any relevant legal aspects. The data base may not be as complete as one wishes or considers necessary. However, this is a reality in many decision-making situations. A claim that there is a lack of data may be used as a cop-out to impede further discussion, to stall the decision-making process, or to refuse to participate in the critical thinking processes required to resolve ethical problems. The following questions are another element of the decision-making process, to be explored as they are appropriate to a given situation:

Reprinted with permission of the Hastings Center Report.[1]

1. Who should be involved in the decision-making process? Who should make the final decision? Why?
2. What criteria should be used—for example, physiological condition only, economic considerations, psychological status, legal considerations, or social and family considerations?
3. What degree of consent should be obtained from the patient or client?
4. What, if any, moral principles are enhanced or negated by proposed choices for action—for example, truth telling, justice, self-determination, or respect for the individual?

Efforts to clarify more ethical decisions and actions in seeking solutions to the dilemmas presented should include determination of underlying values of the people involved. These aspects of decision making are concerned with articulating various ethical approaches that are involved consciously or subconciously in the decision-making process and with identifying the values involved, such as freedom of choice or distributive justice. They should be articulated as part of the process, as they may result in different ethical approaches for action, as for example:

1. The utilitarian approach that seeks the greatest good for the greatest number and focuses primarily on consequences of action—frequently used in justifying administrative decisions made in the health care delivery system.
2. The formalist or deontological approach that is primarily concerned with determination of duties and obligations using moral principles and rules, such as respect for the individual, telling the truth, and avoiding harm.
3. The Rawlsian approach, maintaining that no one should benefit unless all persons benefit from a proposed action, always considering the least fortunate and most vulnerable.

Any one of these ways of thinking about the "right" decision and choice for action(s) in a specific ethical dilemma may come into direct conflict with the traditional medical ethic that says that one should do no harm and one should do all that one can for the individual patient.

Articulation of a position on a given ethical issue or in a specific situation of conflict, whether at the health worker–client level of interaction or at the policy-making level, involves thoughtful, sensitive consideration of all the elements mentioned: the available data base, general questions involved in the decision-making process itself, articulation of the underlying values of the involved individuals, and consideration of ethical positions or approaches. The reader may think of additional dimensions that should enter into the decision-making process about specific ethical dilemmas. Dilemmas may not be resolved immediately through this process, but one can gain increased clarity about areas of agreement and disagreement and more sensitivity to the issues and complexities involved in ethical dilemmas through reflective thinking and discussion. Such discussion may also lead to the possibility that some ethical dilemmas may be prevented in the future through development of institutional or public policy.

CHAPTER 6: RIGHTS AND OBLIGATIONS

Case Study 1

Linda and Bob are both 21 years old. They were married right after finishing high school. Bob works at a local gas station as a mechanic. Linda occasionally works as a cocktail waitress to augment the family income. Both Linda and Bob attend a local community college sporadically. They live in the large second floor apartment in a house owned by Bob's parents, who both work at a local plant. Linda and Bob have a 20-month-old son and a 5-month old daughter, both born prematurely.

Linda made attemps to use the pill as a means of birth control, as she was "not too keen on kids." Bob is very much opposed to any form of birth control, and this has been the source of many arguments between them. He is Catholic and she was brought up a Methodist.

The public health nurse (PHN) knows the family through their contacts with the local health center and has made follow-up home visits after the birth of each child. The PHN has been spending a great deal of time with this family since the birth of the second child because of Linda's hostility and apparent inability to cope with another child. Linda did not want the PHN to come for visits but finally relented when the hospital said these visits were required in order for the baby to go home. At one point during the past year, Linda commented to the nurse that, though she did not want anyone to know, she thought that Bob hurt Billy, the son, when she was working. Billy had bruises on his forehead and thighs, and Bob said that Billy fell off his rocking horse. Linda also mentioned that Bob did not seem very "happy" lately and was recently involved in a fistfight at a local bar. She is afraid that he is abusing alcohol and other drugs.

The PHN knows that there is a state law about reporting suspected child abuse. Then she thinks about the progress that she has been making with Linda and the baby daughter. She also recalls that Linda said no one is to know about her suspicions of Bob.

Further Questions for Discussion

1. What are the ethical problems in this situation?

2. What are the PHN's obligations in this situation to the children, the parents, the agency, the community, and herself? What are the parental obligations?
3. What ethical and moral principles would you consider in reaching a decision? Why?

Case Study 2

John is an "average" high school student on renal dialysis at home. He is 16 years old and started dialysis for the second time after his kidney transplant began to fail. His kidney problems began after a sports injury a few years ago. He is the second oldest of four children. His older sister is in college and two younger brothers are at home. His mother died 2 years ago in an auto accident. John's grandmother, a widow, lives with the family now and is the person responsible for helping him with his dialysis at home. John has a close relationship with both his father and his grandmother. He remained generally optimistic until his transplanted kidney began to fail.

On his last visit to the dialysis center for a periodic checkup, he confided several things to one of the nurses he has known throughout his illness. He claimed he did not want anyone else to know about these things. "I mean it—don't tell anybody; the docs, my dad, or my grandmother—nobody." John was thinking about committing suicide. He had not decided how and wondered if the nurse could do something to help or "maybe I just won't have any more of these treatments." He told the nurse that the reason he wanted to commit suicide was because he knew his dad was having some business problems and might have trouble paying his sister's college tuition. His younger brother needed some orthodontic work. He also knew that his dad planned to remarry and his grandmother would probably leave to live in an apartment. He felt that he would probably die soon. "Why drag it out?" On the other hand, he had just heard about some new research that Dr. S. was doing and thought that maybe he should stay around to participate in it "even if it won't help me."

Further Questions for Discussion

1. What are the ethical problems in this situation?
2. What are the nurse's obligations to John, his family, the physician, and others involved in his care? What are John's rights and obligations?
3. What ethical and moral principles would you consider in reaching a decision? Why?

CHAPTER 7: INFORMED CONSENT

Case Study 1

Mr. S. and his wife have been visiting their 10-year-old daughter, Tina, daily since she was admitted to the hospital four days ago. She has a diagnosis of cancer of the liver, but the parents, who are on welfare, have not been told the diagnosis. The physician feels that the parents, who are Spanish-speaking, will not comprehend any of the terminology necessary to understand the diagnosis. The nurses on the unit have described the parents as "dull" but feel that they should have an explanation of Tina's illness so that they may give the required informed consent for various procedures including some that are experimental. Both Mr. and Mrs. S. have asked the nurses about what is going to happen to Tina. They know that Tina is critically ill.

Further Questions for Discussion

1. What are the elements of the consent process for therapy and for research?
2. What is the nurse's obligation to the parents and to the child to obtain "informed consent?"
3. What ethical and moral principles would you consider in reaching a decision? Why?

Case Study 2

Mrs. R. is a woman in her mid-40s with multiple sclerosis. She has two teen-age daughters, 14 and 16 years old, living at home. Mr. R., a middle-management executive in a local firm, left the home 5 years ago. Mrs. R. often comes into the emergency room of the local community hospital for treatment of acute episodes of asthma. The physician has ordered that if Mrs. R arrests during an acute episode, she is not to be resuscitated. As far as nurses know, the physician made this decision on his own, with no input from the patient or others significant to her or depending on her. One nurse is terribly upset, because this decision conflicts strongly with her own professional and personal moral values. She herself has said on several occasions that Mrs. R.'s home situation is "intolerable" and "I certainly wouldn't want to live under those circumstances." None of the nurses have heard Mrs. R. express any similar feeling about her situation, even though she usually seems somewhat depressed when she comes into the emergency room.

Further Questions for Discussion
1. What are the nurse's obligations in this situation?
2. What ethical and moral principles would you consider in reaching a decision? Why?

CHAPTER 8: ABORTION

Case Study 1

Joan is an 18-year-old pregnant teen-ager who is receiving prenatal care at a local health center. She had a baby last year that she decided to keep with the help of her family, with whom she lives. She has been attending high school and had hoped to graduate next year. However, she dropped out of school recently because she had not been feeling "up to par" with this pregnancy. She works part-time as a cashier at one of the local supermarkets.

You are the nurse practitioner caring for Joan, who told you on her first visit that she had been exposed to rubella three weeks earlier when her little brother and several of his classmates had "the measles." She is just entering the second trimester. You have explained to Joan and her mother the risks to the fetus from this exposure. Her mother wants her to have an abortion, but Joan refuses to have it done, claiming a "right" to have her own child. She and her fiancé, who is HIV infected, are deciding whether they should marry or not before the baby is born.

Further Questions for Discussion
1. What are the ethical problems in this situation?
2. What are the nurse's obligations? What are Joan's obligations?
3. What ethical and moral principles would you consider in reaching a decision? Why?

Case Study 2

Mrs. A. is a 39-year-old woman, pregnant for the first time. Both she and her husband are Jewish. She was married last year for the second time.

Her physician suggested that she should have an amniocentesis because of the increased risk of Down's syndrome with the increased maternal age, as well as the risk of Tay-Sachs disease. Mrs. A. was somewhat reluctant because she and her husband are very excited about this pregnancy, as it will be the first grandchild in each of their families.

Mrs. A. has amniocentesis performed, which shows that the fetus, a female, does have Tay-Sachs disease. The A.s are heartbroken about the situation and are trying to decide whether or not Mrs. A. should have an abortion so that she can become pregnant again as soon as possible.

You are the community health nurse visiting Mrs. A.'s mother, who lives with her daughter after a stroke. Mrs. A. has been discussing her indecision about the abortion with you.

Further Questions for Discussion
1. What are the obligations of the nurse who feels that Mrs. A. should definitely have the abortion?
2. What are the professional health worker's obligations to his or her own personal values in patient interaction?
3. What ethical and moral principles would you consider in reaching a decision? Why?

CHAPTER 9: DYING AND DEATH

Case Study 1
Mr. C., a 48-year-old salesman, arrives on your unit with a "living will" or advance directive to which he has given much thought and attention. He is divorced and remarried and has two children, 9 and 11 years old, from his second marriage. Mr. C. is having a second surgical procedure for cancer of the bowel after surgery and radiation therapy 6 months ago. He has been told by the physician that he has metastasis to the liver and that he should get his affairs in order.

Living wills are legally binding in your state. You do not agree with some of the conditions in Mr. C.'s living will as stated and wonder if you should try to change his mind. You feel that "extraordinary means" should be used because of Mr. C.'s children: "They should have their father with them as long as possible." Mr. C.'s wife has already told you that she thinks a "living will" is totally unnecessary as the "doctors should decide."

Further Questions for Discussion
1. What are the ethical problems in this situation?
2. What are the nurse's obligations? What are the patient's rights and obligations?
3. What ethical and moral principles would you consider in reaching a decision? Why?

Case Study 2
Jack is 14 years old. He was brought into the intensive care unit of the local community hospital after an accident while playing foot-

ball. He has been on a respirator since the accident 2 months ago and is in a persistent vegetative state. Jack's father is manager of a local discount store. His mother is active in church and busy with five other children, all younger than Jack. The youngest has Down's syndrome and attends a special class at the local public school. The nurses know that Jack's hospitalization is a terrible drain on this family, financially and emotionally.

Jack's mother has asked one of the night nurses to "just unplug the the respirator sometime when you're on duty. Who's to know?" The physician has not discussed this with Jack's parents and has adopted a "wait and see" attitude because he knows of a similar case where a patient on a respirator for 8 months is now back in school.

Further Questions for Discussion
1. What are the ethical problems in this situation?
2. Do Jack's siblings and parents have "rights" that should be considered in this situation? Why or why not?
3. What are the nurses' obligations?
4. What ethical and moral principles would you consider in reaching a decision? Why?

CHAPTER 10: BEHAVIOR CONTROL

Case Study 1
Mrs. T. is a 42-year-old woman with a history of occasional depressive episodes. Her husband is a successful businessman in their community. Their third and youngest child is a college freshman in another state. The other children are married. Mrs. T. has her own real estate business, which is moderately successful.

Mrs. T. is a patient in a private psychiatric facility for a third depressive episode in the past 4 years. She has been on various medications, but now her psychiatrist has ordered that she have a series of electric shock treatments (EST). Mrs. T. refuses these treatments and says that there must be something other than EST that the doctor can prescribe.

Further Questions for Discussion
1. What are Mrs. T.'s "rights" in this situation? What are her obligations?
2. What are the nurse's obligations as a patient advocate?
3. Should Mrs. T.'s husband be involved in the decision making that occurs? Why or why not?
4. What ethical and moral principles should you consider in reaching your decisions? Why?

Case Study 2

Bob is an 8-year-old third grader who has been diagnosed as "hyperactive" by his family doctor and put on amphetamines so that he can "quiet down and learn something in school." You are the school nurse and are concerned that Bob did not have a complete psychological or neurological work-up before he started taking the amphetamines his teacher has told you about. You know that Bob's family has had several crisis situations recently—for example, the birth of a new baby and a great-grandfather moving into the home. You feel this makes a complete evaluation for Bob even more critical. You also know that treatment with amphetamines as well as labeling a child "hyperactive" is controversial.

Bob has been an only child until this time and has been described as an average student with "some occasional difficulty in concentrating on his work." Bob's parents both teach school and are very concerned about their son and his academic progress.

Further Questions for Discussion
1. What "rights" do children have to health care?
2. What are some of the problems in ensuring that a child's rights are exercised in the health care system?
3. What are the school nurse's obligations?
4. What ethical and moral principles would you consider in reaching your decision? Why?

CHAPTER 11: MENTAL RETARDATION

Case Study 1

Jane is 19 years old and lives at home with her parents and two "normal" siblings, a brother 16 years old and a sister 9 years old. The father works in a local factory as a foreman. Her mother is at home and cares for Jane's widowed grandmother, who recently moved into the home after surgery for an arthritic hip. Jane has Down's syndrome and is mildly retarded. She goes to a sheltered workshop every day by herself on the bus. She had one out-of-wedlock baby last year, which her parents adopted. They want her to be sterilized, but Jane does not want this done. She insists that she wants to use the pill, which she gets from her family doctor. She continues to have unprotected sex and expressed some concerns about AIDS.

The only contact that the PHN has had recently with Jane is at the bus stop where Jane waits for the local bus. Yesterday Jane mentioned that she had been robbed twice on her way home from the bus stop and that she thinks she might be pregnant. This has not been confirmed and the nurse refrains from asking her if she has thought about an abortion this time, but does suggest that Jane see a physician or the nurse practitioner at the local family planning center.

Further Questions for Discussion
1. What are the ethical problems in this situation?
2. Should the nurse intervene any further? Why or why not?
3. What ethical and moral principles would you consider in reaching your decision? Why?

Case Study 2
The J. family is a family of moderate means with five children. Mr. J. is a long-distance truck driver. Tommy, the youngest child, age 6, has Down's syndrome with moderate retardation and lives in a residential school. He was recently hospitalized for surgery.

Mrs. J. tells the nurses on the surgical unit that she and her husband have had some pressure from the social worker and other staff members of the state residential school to take Tommy back into their home under the policy of deinstitutionalization. Mr. and Mrs. J. find the present arrangement satisfactory, as Mrs. J. also works. They feel that it would be too much of a strain to have Tommy at home again. He was at home for the first year of his life and still needs much supervision. There are community resources available for children of school age, but Mrs. J. would have the major responsibility for Tommy's care at home.

One of the nurses said that she would not want Tommy at home. Another said that she felt that Mr. and Mrs. J. should take him home: "After all, he is their child and he's not as retarded as some others I've seen."

Further Questions for Discussion
1. What are the nurses' obligations to Tommy, to his parents, and to the community? What are the parents' obligations to Tommy and his siblings?
2. What ethical and moral principles would you consider in reaching your decision? Why?

CHAPTER 12: PUBLIC POLICY AND HEALTH CARE DELIVERY

Case Study 1
The nursing director of a community nursing agency has received notice that certain families in the agency case load are no longer eligible for Medicaid funds. These funds have been cut back by authorization of the state. The director has also heard recently that the agency will lose two staff nurse positions as well. Agency funds

set aside for emergency purposes are exhausted. Cost containment continues to be emphasized by the county and state.

All the Medicaid families need continued nursing supervision. The director is also very concerned about the "quality" of nursing care that the nurses can provide in terms of numbers of available staff and the many Medicare patients who continue to increase the agency case load. New referrals for patients on Medicare arrive daily in the agency. These patients require many new high-tech treatments. The nurses are not always prepared to supervise them.

Further Questions for Discussion
1. What are the ethical problems in this situation?
2. What are the director's moral obligations to patients, to staff, to the agency, and to the community?
3. What ethical principles would you consider in reaching your decision(s)? Why?
4. Is the public morally obligated to provide nursing care for everyone needing such care when they have no source of payment? Why or why not?

Case Study 2
You practice nursing in a state reconsidering its existing substance abuse legislation for pregnant women. The law is designed to stop drug use by pregnant women and get them into treatment. Doctors and other health professionals, including nurses, who have evidence that a pregnant woman is using hard drugs are required to report their findings to county child protection workers. The law also requires testing infants after birth if there is reason to believe the mother used controlled substances. A group of nurses in the state has decided to organize and present a position paper on this issue to the legislative committee.

Questions for Discussion
1. What ethical principles might be considered in looking at proposed changes in the legislation?
2. What public values are expressed in the present legislation?
3. With what private values held by individuals, families, or health professionals might these public values conflict?
4. Write a proposed piece of legislation to deal with this issue that is ethically justifiable.

REFERENCE

1. Callahan D: Values, facts and decision making. *Hastings Cent Rep* 6:1, June 1971.

Index